NEUROLOGY - LABORATORY AND CLINICAL RESEARCH DEVELOPMENTS

ASPERGER SYNDROME

RISK FACTORS, COGNITIVE-BEHAVIORAL CHARACTERISTICS AND MANAGEMENT STRATEGIES

NEUROLOGY - LABORATORY AND CLINICAL RESEARCH DEVELOPMENTS

Additional books in this series can be found on Nova's website
under the Series tab.

Additional e-books in this series can be found on Nova's website
under the e-book tab.

NEUROLOGY - LABORATORY AND CLINICAL RESEARCH DEVELOPMENTS

ASPERGER SYNDROME

RISK FACTORS, COGNITIVE-BEHAVIORAL CHARACTERISTICS AND MANAGEMENT STRATEGIES

MICHAEL F. SHAUGHNESSY
EDITOR

NOVA BIOMEDICAL

New York

Library of Congress Cataloging-in-Publication Data

ISBN: 978-1-63463-810-4

Library of Congress Control Number: 2014958720

Published by Nova Science Publishers, Inc. † New York

Contents

Introduction

The syndrome, the condition, the nomenclature surrounding Asperger's Syndome has been around for decades. It is been studied, research, written about and discussed. Recently, there has been a move to eliminate Asperger's from the latest Diagnostic and Statistical Manual of the American Psychiatric Association. This has caused some concern, discussion and consternation in various quarters. Questions have been raised and clinicians are bracing for the ramifications and repercussions of such as decision.

Those impacted are those who have been diagnosed or labeled with Asperger's years ago. Their identity, their being and their essence has been defined and explained by this label. It has provided some understanding and a certain amount of validation to those impacted.

This book will attempt to delve into some of the main relevant realms regarding Asperger's. Worldwide, there are nations in which Asperger's is still the diagnosis of choice, and there are nations in which teachers and counselors are working with students that are formally diagnosed, and continue to be labeled as Asperger's.

Some of the chapters will address language and speech issues. Some of the chapters will address inter-personal and familial issues, and some will address management issues of girls and boys in the school systems in various countries (England, Australia etc.).

There are humanistic papers that address the strengths and weaknesses of all human beings and the need to address these areas. New advances in neurofeedback and electrical imaging will be examined. Some clinical tools such as the Quick Protocol for Pragmatic Assessment will be explored.

Lastly, a parent and teacher's perspective on Asperger's will be offered summarizing the human element in this realm. This text is by no means a comprehensive review of all of the issues. There are vocational, cognitive, and other issues that will need to be explored by other scholars in the future. There may be new advances in medicine and other realms which may shed more light into the mysterious condition that is now considered to be " high functioning autism " rather than a distinct entity such as Asperger's Syndrome. For those who are working with children, adolescents, and adults with Asperger's – we salute you and your efforts. For those previously diagnosed and now grappling with these changes, we understand and support you and hope that you are validated in the future.

Certainly, more resources are needed and more counseling services need to be provided for both those diagnosed with Asperger's as well as the teachers who have to provide instruction and the parents who have to prepare them for the world of adulthood and work. It is hoped that this book is a step in the right direction.

Dr. Michael F. Shaughnessy, Editor
Professor, Eastern New Mexico University,
School of Education
Portales, New Mexico, US
Michael.Shaughnessy@enmu.edu

In: Asperger Syndrome
Editor: Michael F. Shaughnessy

ISBN: 978-1-63463-810-4

Chapter 1

Asperger Syndrome and the Perils of Pluto

Michael F. Shaughnessy**, *June Shepherd and Danielle Jackovitz
Eastern New Mexico University, NM, US

Abstract

Recently, the revision of the Diagnostic and Statistical Manual resulted in the dropping of the diagnosis or disorder of what was formerly referred to as Asperger Syndrome. Those individuals that had been diagnosed or labeled as being Asperger's will now receive a diagnosis of "High Functioning Autism." This paper will examine and explore the implications of this change. This paper will discuss the therapeutic issues surrounding the adjustment of those previously diagnosed as Asperger Syndrome and will review the concerns of parents, peers and family members regarding this re-alignment of DSM- 5. Some of the tangential concerns will be addressed and explored.

Keywords: Asperger Syndrome, high functioning autism, DSM-V

Introduction

The diagnosis of Asperger's has been around for quite some time. It stems from the work of Hans Asperger who identified a cluster of symptoms, behaviors, speech and language differences and idiosyncratic verbalizations. This paper will review a bit of the history of Asperger's and discuss first its inclusion in the Diagnostic and Statistical Manuals, and its recent removal from the DSM. The implications of this will be discussed in terms of insurance, treatment, behavioral issues and cognitive assessment, as well as counseling issues

* Corresponding author: Michael.Shaughnessy@enmu.edu.

for those previously diagnosed as "Asperger Syndrome" who now have to re-adjust to a new labeling and nomenclature- one with which they may not be entirely comfortable.

The backdrop to this will be the perils of Pluto. As many scientists, teachers and others know, Pluto was considered a planet for many years. However, recently, Pluto was re-categorized and is no longer considered a "planet", causing great consternation and a good deal of adjustment for many textbook writers and astronomers. Obviously "Pluto" continues in the solar system above, and it is somewhat disconcerting to hear that it is no longer a planet, but some other body of rock in the solar system. While the orbiting mass of rock may not care what it is called, there is consternation on the part of science teachers, parents, children and others and those in the field to have these kinds of frivolous changes occur.

A Bit of History

Hans Asperger first wrote about the condition which now bears his name in the year 1944. Hans Asperger was able to observe normal intelligibility among children who displayed autistic-like behaviors including a lack of social skills. When Asperger's was included in APA's Diagnostic and Statistical Manuel of Mental Disorders (DSM-V) it was clearly distinct from Autism. Asperger's has been recognized as a health condition for over 60 years and society has only just begun to understand the social and psychological impact that it has on those with the diagnosis. In order to offer useful support for this population, we must learn what the diagnosis really means. We must learn what it means to the family and to the individual diagnosed with this disorder or syndrome. Obviously, much has been written about Asperger Syndrome and the entire realm of literature and research will not be reviewed here. We will however, endeavor to examine and explore some of the main issues and discuss some of the salient concerns.

On occasion, a group of individuals gets together to reevaluate and reassess the various psychiatric conditions and mental health and developmental difficulties encountered by psychiatrists, psychologists, and neurologists and others in the field. Certainly, the first Diagnostic and Statistical Manual is quite different from the one that exists today, as we have become more aware of various conditions, and as research has been conducted and case studies investigated.

A group of professionals in the field were recently charged with the revision of the DSM-IV-TR and the result was the DSM-5, (Diagnostic and Statistical Manual-5th Edition) which is now available to the general public.

The revision of the DSM-V was headed by David Kupfer, M.D. and he has attempted to clarify why the change occurred.

DSM-5's revised diagnosis of autism spectrum disorder is a more accurate and medically and scientifically useful way of diagnosing autism-related disorders. Using DSM-IV, patients could be diagnosed with four separate disorders: autistic disorder, Asperger Syndrome disorder, childhood disintegrative disorder, and the catch-all diagnosis of pervasive developmental disorder not otherwise specified. Researchers found that these separate diagnoses were not consistently applied across different clinics and treatment centers and really represented symptoms and behaviors along a severity continuum, rather than distinct disorders. Anyone who was diagnosed with one of the four disorders using DSM-IV should still meet the criteria for autism spectrum disorder or another diagnosis using DSM-5 (Shaughnessy, Arrington, Dawson, West, and Harrell, 2014)

The Re-Adjustment Issues

Since "Asperger's" has been formally removed from DSM-V, there has been some concern about those who were previously diagnosed with this terminology. Their identity, their existence, their being, has been that of a person with "Asperger Syndrome." For many people, the diagnosis provides an anchor of sorts to help them understand the reactions of others and to comprehend their difficulties with interpersonal relations and social difficulties.

In psychiatry and various other fields, the use of a diagnosis often provides some relief to a patient. When a doctor indicates to a patient that they have, for example, hyperpyrexia, there is a sigh of relief in that there is now a word, a label that hopefully will lead to treatment. This has often been referred to by various names as the Rumpelstilitskin effect, although there are other frames of reference to explain this phenomenon. A diagnosis, for some people provides an explanation as to why things are the way they are, and provides an "anchor" of sorts to help in understanding why they behave the way they do. For example, once a person is diagnosed with Parkinson's for example, they begin a long process that may lead to treatment and or recovery. It may lead to some grasp of understanding as to why they have been feeling, acting, thinking, in a certain way.

The Impact of the Deletion of "Asperger Syndrome"

Although one would question exactly how many individuals are diagnosed with Asperger Syndrome around the world, there probably are ramifications and repercussion for many individuals.

a) For those previously diagnosed – They may be in a state of shock, dismay, disbelief. Their world has been turned upside down, and they begin to perhaps question the medical profession. They begin to question the world of psychiatry.
b) For those whose identify is clearly that of an individual with Asperger Syndrome. These individuals may have a clear specific idea of themselves as a certain group or subgroup. They may have been to a support group and have received validation, support and encouragement as well as acceptance.
c) Support for those in adjustment – For those who may have just been recently diagnosed, these individuals may need some supportive therapy as they begin to readjust to a new diagnosis. While this may not be seen as a major factor for those not in the field, for those grasping for understanding, this is a precarious adjustment.
d) Emotional Issues regarding the change – Any change is stressful. A change in one's identity, a change in one's self perception and other perception is an emotionally draining experience. A fully formed identity may be ripped to shreds as the person has to adjust to another diagnosis. A caring competent counselor may continue to

treat the person, with their adjustment and emotional concerns, and not become preoccupied with the diagnostic nosology and nomenclature.

e) Massive change and shift in textbooks – For textbook authors, for psychology instructors, the change may be a challenge. They may have to decide how to reconcile this change with previous texts or literature.

f) World wide – We do not know what the change will bring about and what will they do in other counties in terms of this change. It may take quite a while for the change to impact the field, other therapists and individuals who manifest some of the behaviors of those diagnosed as Asperger Syndrome in the past.

g) Clients, patients, parents will all be summarily impacted by the change. One wonders how do we explain to patients/clients previously diagnosed with Asperger Syndrome about this change? How will this impact various support groups? What will be their agendas? What will be the over-arching concerns?

h) Overall, for some the change may seem minor and insignificant. For others, this is a major shift in thinking, treatment, diagnosis, and nomenclature. Just as scientists were upset when Pluto was no longer deemed a planet, many individuals are upset that Asperger Syndrome- a syndrome studied for years, has now been changed to something entirely different, at least in the minds of some people and clinicians.

For more than 19 years (1994-2013), several million people in the United States and around the world received the neurodevelopmental diagnosis known as Asperger Syndrome from physicians, psychiatrists, psychologists, and other mental health professionals. The ages ranged from early childhood to middle age or older for adults. Although the diagnosis always included normal to high intelligence and normal language development in childhood, they have what observers would describe as very noticeable deficits in social interactions with others and odd, repetitive patterns of behaviors, interests, and activities. For so many years, they were considered by the general public as being odd, eccentric, immature, or just plain weird. Being misunderstood in this way was very painful and difficult for those with Asperger Syndrome and their family members. Most with Asperger Syndrome wanted to fit in and not stand out but because of their neurological problems; they suffered serious deficits that prevented them from knowing how to be what they and others would call "normal."

Most of what the general public knew about Asperger Syndrome , they learned through watching TV shows such as Boston Legal, Parenthood, and The Big Bang Theory and movies such as Adam and Mozart and the Whale and others. The characters portrayed with Asperger Syndrome were very true to life. They had normal to high intelligence and had normal language development but as mentioned before, they had serious problems relating to others and had some unusual, noticeable, and odd behaviors. Sometimes they talked incessantly and in great detail about certain subjects that others weren't interested in, or, would talk too loud or too softly in a monotone voice. Sometimes, they would have no eye contact at all, would stand way too close to someone when talking to them, or would laugh when others were sad.

Some would engage in odd self-stimulatory behaviors such flapping their hands, rocking back and forth, or they had difficulty organizing their belongings, completing tasks, or were fanatic about sticking to daily routines that they repeated over and over. They would became upset and disoriented if anything or person tried to interrupt their routines. They had great difficulty understanding jokes and were very gullible. Typically, they were only interested in talking about their subjects of interest and could not read facial expressions when others were bored with them and wanted them to stop talking. Some also exhibited trouble understanding when and what, to keep private.

Through the characters portrayed, we also learned to appreciate other very endearing qualities about people with Asperger Syndrome such as; being loyal and sensitive, having a gentle soul, being worthy of trust, being a good worker, sometimes a good provider, being faithful, as well as having lots of talents. Many have a great sense of humor, and can be very sweet and polite. The social media exposure promoted compassion and understanding for the disorder. Most importantly, persons with Asperger Syndrome were validated and felt respected and they saw through the actors and in each other, a potential for living life with Asperger Syndrome in new and inspiring ways. For the first time, they saw themselves as not that far off from normal.

Over the years, especially the last ten, people diagnosed with Asperger Syndrome began to identify deeply with their label of Asperger's Syndrome. The diagnosis evolved into cultural nicknames such as "Aspies, Aspergians, Aspergirls, and even Asperkids ." The nicknames became a social moniker, something considered desirable and symbolizing a form of acceptance. The label helped persons with Asperger's to find each other, develop camaraderie with fellow "Aspies", as well as comfort and learning from each other. They found a place that welcomed them. They found a place where they belonged, which in turn, resulted in unprecedented self-care and self-understanding for many.

Online support groups and chat rooms for "Aspies" helped to connect "Aspies" all over the world. Numerous advocacy groups were created and still exist. Many benefited from the numerous services provided through public schools, trainings for parents, therapy and support groups. Books were written for "Aspies" to help them during their college years, with dating relationships and even marriage counseling. A whole new world of possibility for their futures was opened up for them. Being an "Aspie" had in some ways become "cool."

A lot of clinical information was gathered from 1994 to 2013. The scholars and researchers, who compiled the research during the last few decades, changed their minds. They concluded that the criteria for a diagnosis of Asperger's should be updated and modified. Through their research, they determined that Asperger's was really on the high functioning end of what is referred to as The Autism Spectrum. They were saying that Asperger Syndrome was a form of autism separated only by levels of severity of the disorder and they decided that the previous label, Asperger Syndrome, was no longer an appropriate diagnostic label. That happened in May of 2013 and many people have been in an uproar ever since. No more Asperger's? What?!?! There was consternation and confusion and chaos all around!

Before there was time for clarifications and explanations to get to the public as a whole, there was an immediate and intense reaction from the Asperger's community. People were mad and hurt. They did not like people outside of the "Aspie" community making such life altering decisions about their lives!

Many thought that they were being told that "their" Asperger Syndrome problems didn't exist anymore and that people were trying to just get rid of them.

Some worried about not getting covered by insurance if they were now considered "autistic." Some welcomed the merging of Asperger Syndrome and Autistic communities while others felt embarrassed being that closely associated with people with Autism, who they thought were so much worse off than people with Asperger Syndrome. The way people with Asperger Syndrome talked about autism, hurt the feelings of many diagnosed as autistic.

Others expressed concern that now that they had improved a lot, they might not be "bad enough" to qualify for autism services under the new guidelines. It was as if their identity as someone with Asperger Syndrome was being ripped from them. Many began to retreat, withdraw, and grieve. They had so deeply identified with Asperger's, and it seemed it was now being taken away from them. Many expressed anxiety, depression, and hopelessness and – it should be noted that one of the hallmark characteristics of persons with Asperger Syndrome is that they hate change!

Andrew Solomon, author of *Far From the Tree,* helps us understand why so many people with the previous diagnosis of Asperger's feel threatened and vulnerable about losing their identity as an "Aspie." He explained the threat as a result of a person having more of a "horizontal than vertical identity."

He explains that most people define their identity as a combination of their religion, their race, their language and nationality. Those are called "vertical identities." Vertical identities are like a conduit through which the benefits of shared life experience such as empathy and hindsight, and a sense of who we are, can travel or glow from generation to generation to generation.

But let's suppose you are born with schizophrenia or are deaf or have a serious physical disability and your parents have none of those problems. Let's say you are a child prodigy, you were born out of rape, or you were highly gifted and talented or born with Asperger Syndrome and your parents had none of those experiences. People born with such conditions identify more with what some would call their illness, their affliction, or their flaw. Those identities are considered "horizontal identities." A horizontal identity occurs when there is a rupture between the child's life experiences and the parents' experiences. People with "horizontal identities" are often an embarrassment and a disappointment to their family. The person with the horizontal identity often is seen as challenging and interrupting the basic continuity of the family they are born into. Through Solomon's research, he discovered that when a child's identity falls far outside the family's identity, there seems to be a non-transferable sympathy between the family and the child.

Concerns About This DSM–V Change

One major concern indicated by parents is that their son or daughter's treatment for Asperger Syndrome may no longer be covered by Insurance. There is concern that services may be cut. There is concern that services that are needed may not continue. Some are adamant about keeping the label of "Asperger Syndrome."

Treatments/Therapies

While some have accepted the nomenclatural change and the shift in psychiatric nosology, there has been little forthcoming in terms of treatment options and alternatives. Perhaps future textbooks by those working in the field will indicate the new different treatment options and alternatives for those individuals now seen as "high functioning autistic" as opposed to those previously labeled as Asperger Syndrome. Perhaps other nations in the English speaking world will continue pretty much as they have in the past, ignoring the new DSM-V. Perhaps other clinicians will simply treat the person, the individual and their adjustment and social and vocational problems rather than the diagnosis.

Textbook changes in the future may help those with, and without High Functioning Autism understand and respect each other. At the current time, textbooks across the United States will have to be changed to reflect the deletion of "Asperger Syndrome " and those who were trained in clinical programs years ago, will have to make certain adjustments. For those trained in decades past, the adjustment may not be traumatic or extensive. Certainly some remember the diagnosis of "Minimal Brain Dysfunction" which was the precursor of "Attention Deficit Disorder." Going back centuries, many thought that epilepsy and seizures were caused by demonic possession. Certainly nowadays, we do not see this as appropriate. We now know that seizures are caused by random electrical firing in the brain and not some demon or devil.

World Wide Changes

As these changes have been somewhat recent, it is too soon to ascertain the impact of the DSM-V changes in other English Speaking countries, although with e-mail, it is increasingly easy to communicate with other clinicians who work with children and adolescents and adults who have been diagnosed as Asperger Syndrome and remain diagnosed as Asperger Syndrome. Research continues in England, Australia, and other English speaking countries, and some of that research is included in this text. It is not clear if the International Classification of Diseases will go along with DSM-V as I.C.D. (International Classification of Diseases) may be seen by many as the standard for all mental disorders.

Even with the Internet, change comes slowly. Some clinicians are resistant to change, and some adhere to older anachronistic methods.

Summary and Conclusion

This chapter has attempted to provide an overview of the issue regarding the deletion of Asperger Syndrome from the DSM-5. It has discussed some of the concerns and areas to be explored and examined. The other chapters in the book will supplement this chapter, delving into great depth and detail some of the salient domains in this realm.

References

American Psychiatric Association: Diagnostic and Statistical Manual of Mental Disorders, Fifth Edition. Arlington, VA, American Psychiatric Association, 2013.

Shaughnessy, M.F., Arington, T., Dawson, L., West, L.& Harrell, L. (2014) An Interview with David Kupfer. *North American Journal of Psychology.* 16, 2, 235-241.

In: Asperger Syndrome
Editor: Michael F. Shaughnessy

ISBN: 978-1-63463-810-4

Chapter 2

Sensory Regulation for Inclusive Classrooms

Kara Collyer and Ingrid Harrington *

University of New England, Australia

Abstract

Sensory integration (SI) theory and therapy, and sensory integration based therapies (SIB), are relatively new concepts in the field of education and occupational therapy, to better improve the inclusion of students with sensory processing dysfunction in education classrooms, specifically those diagnosed on the Autistic Spectrum with Asperger Syndrome (Devlin et al., 2010). Practitioners and parents report benefits of sensory integration interventions in various areas: maintaining attention, higher levels of cognition activity, and improved social skills and self-stimulating behaviours (Devlin et al., 2010; Yack, Aquila and Sutton, 2002). This chapter reviews current literature in these fields from a perspective on how these theories and therapies can improve the inclusion of students with ASD in educational settings.

Keywords: Sensory processing, sensory integration, sensory integration based interventions, Asperger Syndrome

Introduction

Approximately 80 studies within the past five years have reported the impact implementing sensory integration approaches have on the improvement of learning and engagement to students with special learning needs in an inclusive education classroom (Yack et al., 2002). Despite the promise these theories and therapies can offer these students with special learning needs, the larger scale effectiveness and impact of the approaches on the

* Corresponding author: Ingrid Harrington. E-mail: iharring@une.edu.au.

complete classroom cohort have been deemed inconclusive due to the small-scale size of the research samples. Therefore a lack of research exists in reporting the benefits and/or drawbacks of implementing the same inclusive sensory regulation program that is inclusive of *all* students in the mainstream classroom.

To understand holistically how sensory integration and SI and SIB interventions work, an understanding first of what sensory processing is, how sensory processing effects learning, and the symptoms of an unregulated sensory system will be explored. Sensory integration therapy and sensory integration based interventions will be outlined including who will most benefit from sensory integration therapy, and what may be the possible benefits of implementing a whole class sensory regulation program in an education classroom.

Due to the lack of research reporting the impact of a whole class sensory program, and fewer in the area of sensory based integration therapy (Yack et al., 2002), it needs to be noted that the literature reviewed focused on individuals and small groups, with most data being collected from parents and therapists. This chapter will explore the design and impact of an inclusive sensory regulation program to be used in a mainstream education classroom. A sensory regulation program for an inclusive classroom should have an educational approach, with the data being collected from teacher reports, academic progress, engagement and the effect on anti-social behaviour.

What Is Sensory Processing and How Does It Affect Learning?

Humphrey (2002, p. 172) describes sensory processing as the "registration and modulation of sensory information [and the] internal organisation of sensory input." Sensory processing allows human beings to execute successful adaptive responses to situational demands that allow meaningful engagement in daily life. Adaptive behaviours are purposeful and enable the individual to overcome challenges and to learn new skills (Prudhomme White et al., 2007).

Sensory processing is a function of the nervous system that receives, organises and understands sensory information from both our bodies and environmental inputs (Smith Myles et al., 2001). Effective sensory processing is vital for everyone to engage and fully participate in daily roles and routines such as learning (Huebner and Dunn, 2001; Jenkinson, Hyde and Ahmad, 2008). Sensory processing has been broken down into seven categories that are all integrated and linked with each other. They include the Vestibular, Proprioceptive, Tactile, Auditory, Visual, Olfactory and Gustatory (Smith Myles et al. 2000). Vestibular, Proprioceptive and Tactile are the main foundation sensory systems included in the inclusive classroom sensory regulation program that will be the focus later in this chapter. Activities that are planned to regulate vestibular, proprioceptive and tactile, have the most effect on regulation of the sensory system by, lasting the longest and activities being able to be altered to different speeds to regulate an underactive or overactive sensory system (Culp, 2011; Yack et al., 2002). As reflected in Figure 1, the tactile, vestibular and proprioceptive systems are the foundation upon which learning is reliant.

Dunn (1997, pg. 24) developed a model of sensory processing characteristics that include: low registration, sensation seeking, sensory sensitivity and sensation avoiding. Dunn (1999) also produced a 'sensory profile' that comprised a questionnaire that could be used to determine what sensory characteristics a person exhibits, and therefore allowed interventions to be matched accordingly.

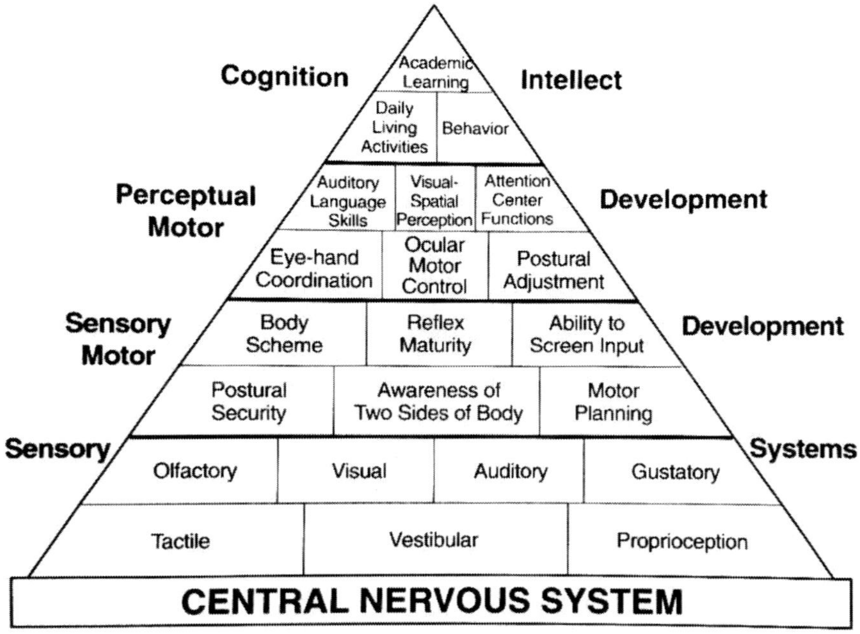

Figure 1. Taylor and Trott, 1991, Cited Williams and Shellenberger, 1994, pg. 4.

"Dunn's Sensory Profile" (Dunn, 1999) made screening for sensory issues easier in children (Scaff and Miller, 2005), yet McIntosh et al. (1999) in the same year developed 'The Short Sensory Profile' based on Dunn's original model. McIntosh's model was far shorter and less time consuming, and for the purposes of the design of an inclusive sensory regulation program, "The Short Sensory Profile" is an essential planning tool.

Who Is at Risk of Sensory Processing Difficulties?

Dunn (2001) provided evidence that linked sensory processing difficulty with numerous genetic and developmental disorders, brain disorders, schizophrenia and chronic fatigue. Devlin, et al's research (2010) focused on children with developmental disabilities, yet eighty to ninety per cent of children with an ASD had been reported to have some type of sensory modulation issue (Baranek, 2002; Huebner, 2001; Kientz and Dunn, 1997; O'Neill and Jones, 1997). Self-regulation, or modulation, are the ways in which our sensory input is managed, but problems occur when there is a difficulty initially responding to sensory input. Dysfunctions in the sensory processing system can be referred to as "Sensory Processing Disorder" or a "Sensory Modulation Disorder" (Watling et al. 2011). Ayres (1979) and Ahn et al. (2004) reported that 5-15% of the whole population has a sensory processing dysfunction, and Roberts et al. (2007) concluded that as much as 20% of students without a disability, will experience some form of sensory dysfunction.

Implications of Sensory Processing Disorder (SPD) and Sensory Moducaiton Disorder (SMD) on Learning

Ayres (1979, p. 51) described sensory dysfunction as "the brain is not processing or organising the flow of sensory impulses in a manner that gives the individual good, precise, sensory input, and not directing behaviour effectively."

When sensory processing lacks efficiency, the function, social interaction, learning and ability to keep ourselves calm and alert becomes a challenge every second of the day (Mailloux and Roley Smith, 2010). When the brain is unable to make sense of sensory input, the person will experience sensory dysfunction.

An individual that experiences sensory dysfunction will experience inconsistencies in their daily functioning performance, and these can vary daily depending upon environmental factors, expectations and mood (Murray-Slutsky and Paris, 2002).

Parham and Mailloux (2005) reported that sensory processing problems are often associated with poor social skills, immature play skills, self-concept, decreased motor skills and participating in daily living skills. Watling et al. (2006) agreed with Parham and Mailloux, (2005) but added descriptions of flawed sensory processing effects upon classroom behaviour, which included not following classroom rules and inappropriately interacting with peers. Dunn (1997, p. 40) suggested the following about children:

- sensory seekers display 'on the move' behaviour;
- sensory avoiders are reluctant to move and withdraw;
- sensory sensitivity children that are easily irritated or distracted are having difficulty processing sensory input; and,
- Low registration students have difficulty paying attention and may seem uninterested.

Students that experience difficulty processing sensory input, may encounter difficulty regulating their activity levels, mood and behaviour. Children need to be taught how to regulate their sensory system in order to be able to self-regulate their emotions, behaviour and reactions (Kuypers, 2013; Williams and Shellenburger, 1994). Inappropriate behaviour may occur because the sensory processing responses are inconsistent to the demand of the situation. Teachers may view this behaviour as 'bad', but a student with sensory processing issues often cannot control these behaviours that teachers refer to as "bad", "anti social" or "negative" (Smith Myles et al. 2001). Grandin (1995, p. 39) eloquently restated that "All the behaviour modification in the world is not going to stop a child from screaming if the sound of the bell hurts."

A study conducted by Gourley et al. (2012) used "The Short Sensory Profile" with 59 parents of preschool children, and reported that 59% of children had sensory processing difficulties. They hypothesized that sensory processing issues were linked with behavioral problems and levels of parental stress.

The study suggested that children that rated higher in sensory processing difficulties also had higher levels of behavioral issues. Their findings lead to discussions that concluded that in order to best address the sensory difficulties in children with behavioral problems, the creating of a successful intervention strategy was the most important step.

Sensory Integration (SI)

Sensory integration is a theory and treatment method developed by Dr. Jean Ayres (1972, 1979), a psychologist and occupational therapist involved in the field of neuroscience. Most of the research in SI and sensory processing is based upon Ayres' Sensory Integration theory (Baranek, 2002; Biel and Peske, 2009; Howe et al., 2004; Milloux and Smith Roley, 2010; Murray-Slutsky and Paris, 2000; Watling et al., 2006; Watling et al., 2011; Williams and Shellenberger, 1994). Ayres (1972, 1979) documented patterns of sensory input processing dysfunction amongst children with learning disabilities. These sensory dysfunctions impact upon motor skills, language, behaviour, cognition and emotional well-being. Ayres (1979, p. 5) introduced the "Theory of Sensory Integration" and defined it as "the organization of the senses for use." In simple terms, SI is the relationship between sensation, brain function and behaviour (Watling et al., 2011). Ayres (1972, 1979) explored further how sensory processing occurred, and found that the higher cognitive parts of the brain, e.g., the prefrontal cortex, are dependent upon the integration and integrity of the information from the senses in order to behaviour "normally." Multiple functions of the brain are impacted neurologically by the integration of sensory information. Emotions and behaviour are directly influenced, as these are processed in the same part of the brain that sensory input is organised, therefore, these impact on each other and the ability of the person to self-regulate.

Key Research

Many researchers have expanded upon and further developed Ayres' Sensory Integration theory. Wilson et al. (1992, p. 27) likened Sensory Integration Treatment to "one-on-one" tutoring and found the results indicated that there was "no difference in academic achievement in both groups", that supports Ayres' theory. Some research reported that SI treatment does affect academic functioning (Baranek 2002, pg. 406, Case-Smith et al., 2001; Oetter et al., 1993). Walting et al. (2011) completed a systematic review of literature addressing evidence-based interventions for children and adolescents with challenges in sensory processing that were published between 1996 and 2008. They concluded that despite a low power in most studies, there was a trend towards positive evidence to support the sensory integration approach.

Oetter et al. (1993) defined "arousal level" as an impact of the sensory system: a person's arousal level will depend upon the situational demands and influence their ability to attend and concentrate. Williams and Shellenberger (1994) added that one must be in an optimal state of arousal to successfully meet the demands of the task, and to do this, one must be able to self-regulate. Oetter et al. (1993) suggested that sensory input must be met to satisfy each individual sensory need, in order for them to reach an appropriate arousal level that is needed for attention and ability to learn. If a person has sensory processing issues, then they would require more or less sensory input to ensure optimal arousal is achieved, and the "Zone of Proximal Development" is targeted (Bodrova and Leong, 2005).

The ability to integrate sensory information is one source that accounts for differences in self-regulation in individuals (Ayres, 1979; Dunn, 1997). Self-regulation is a person's ability to regulate their responses to specific stimuli.

Poor self-regulation skills may increase aggressive behaviours, off task behaviour and low cognitive outcomes (Roberts et al., 2007). Bundy Lane and Murray (2002) added the ability to self-regulate decreased social skills, impaired self-confidence, and diminished motor and sensor motor skill development. Sensory integration therapy was designed to address the underlying neurophysiological processing of sensory input, and requires advanced knowledge and practical skills such as a qualified Occupational Therapist. However, sensory-based interventions can be used in all other areas of the person's life, and these are referred to as sensory integration based interventions (Smith Roley et al., 2009).

Sensory Based Interventions

Sensory-based interventions aim to focus a person's attention and promote acceptable behaviour in schools, home and the community (Baranek, 2002; Watling et al., 2011). They can be facilitated by educators or parents under the recommendations of a sensory integration professional (Smith Roley et al., 2009). Sensory integration-based programs nourish the sensory system and provide the individual with input that relieves the nervous system from "survival mode", and regulates it into a more calm, organised and alert state. Regulation of the sensory system is fundamental to our sense of well-being and the ability to function and learn through daily life (Biel and Peske, 2009; Zeidler, 2012).

Key Research

Wilbarger (1995) developed the term "Sensory diet", which is a sensory integration-based approach used to facilitate a child's ability to keep an alert, organised and calm state. Sensory diets can be implemented in an inclusive classroom without the need of specialised equipment, one-on-one directions, or an Occupational Therapist (Baranek, 2002; Biel and Peske, 2009). Smith Myles et al. (2001) reviewed the effectiveness of occupational therapy practice for children with ASD to get them into a more alert, organised and calm state. The review only used studies that were experimental in design and, when available, synthesized review and meta-analyses where used. Two of the five categories used were sensory focused (SI and SIB), and Smith Myles (2001) concluded that SI and SIB were positive, but effects sizes were small and more rigorous trials were needed.

Vargas and Camilli (1999) published a meta-analysis of research on sensory integration treatment: 27 studies from 1972–1994 where included. Early studies showed that sensory integration treatment approaches were the most effective in achieving an alert, organised and calm state in students. They concluded that the sensory integration intervention was as effective to alternative interventions. They also noted the limitations in methodology of the studies. A qualitative study by Cohn (2000) reported on parents' perceptions of sensory-based interventions, and how they impacted upon the quality of their family life. The results of the study showed that parents saw positive outcomes of sensory integration therapy in three domains of their children's functions: abilities, activities and sense of self-worth.

Scaaf and Nightlinger (2007) used a case study approach to explore the use of sensory integration and their findings report that sensory integration therapy improves the ability to integrate sensory input that influences adaptive behaviour and occupational performance. Baranek (2002) reviewed 13 studies that used either Sensory Integration (SI) therapy or Sensory Integration based interventions (Sensory diet, Touch pressure, Vestibular, exercise and touch therapy) as interventions for children with an ASD, and concluded that all studies had positive outcomes for the individuals. Baranek (2002) reported that the SI and SIB interventions decreased anxiety, improved behaviour, motor skills, self-stimulation and social interactions in the participants. All 13 studies indicated no negative effects upon any individual, therefore, deeming the interventions safe.

Case-Smith et al. (2011) compiled a table of Occupational Therapy focus areas in school-based practice. The table listed 30 goals, such as participation in education, attention, on-task behaviour, academic skills, motor skills and positive behaviour. Each goal coincided with an education outcome followed by providing evidence from SI related research.

Inclusive Practices

Authentic inclusion is determined by personalising learning for all students, making learning relevant and reflective of student's needs, interests and abilities (Lynch and Irvine, 2007). Students in the UK with special educational needs (SEN) are to be educated in mainstream schools with typically developing peers. Humphrey and Lewis (2008, p. 138) reported that a gap between "inclusion rhetoric and classroom reality was very wide in some schools", and that the number of students with an ASD attending mainstream UK schools had risen significantly in the past decade.

Frederickson, Jones and Lang (2010) provided more concrete figures by explaining that between 1997 and 2001, students diagnosed with an ASD more than doubled and the majority of these students were receiving education in mainstream UK schools. Similar figures were also reported in other countries around the world (Glennon, 2010; Leblanc et al., 2009). Research by Mailloux and Roley (2011) indicated that 80-100% of students with an ASD had a sensory processing dysfunction, therefore, education settings needed to be inclusive and support these students' needs for them to be able to fully participate in learning activities. Devlin et al. (2010) reported that 82% of Occupational Therapists always used a sensory integration approach when working with children with ASD. Symptoms of ASD typically include a poor attention span, emotional distress, challenging behaviours, academic difficulties and social challenges (Wilkinson, 2007). The symptoms of SPD, including, but not limited to: challenges in, social skills, fine motor and emotional regulation (Smith Myles et al., 2001) are very similar to ASD, and the two seem to overlap. If the numbers of students with ASD are on the rise and are being educated in mainstream UK classrooms, it would make sense to introduce a sensory based integration program into the daily classroom routine to meet their broad range of needs.

It is the responsibility of educators to put in place strategies for all students to be able to learn among friends, build social relationships and establish a high self-esteem (Lynch and Irvine, 2009). By providing an inclusive sensory regulation program, individual students are not singled out and excluded, thereby, not socially isolated from peers. Lynch and Irvine (2009) summarised several studies that all indicated the implementation of an inclusive sensory regulation program in the classroom had positive effects on students.

Peer acceptance, self-esteem, social skills, engagement, on-task time and positive behaviour all increased as a result of the inclusive practices embedded in the inclusive sensory regulation program (Lynch and Irvine, 2009). Grey et al. (2007) also concluded that inclusive practices increased social acceptance, on task behaviour and academic achievement. Chandler-Olcott and Kluth (2009) reported that inclusive education was beneficial for all involved, not just the SEN student, showing positive effects on the classroom community as a whole.

Supporting students in mainstream classrooms with ASD is challenging but can be successfully achieved if appropriate supports are in place (Wilkinson, 2007). A sensory regulation program that includes an inclusive whole class "sensory diet" would be seen as an appropriate support for students with an ASD, and many other students who may have sensory processing difficulties. Lynch and Irvine's (2009, p. 853) comprehensive review of literature on best practice for children with ASD, recommended that "integrating ASD-specific education supports with a general inclusive education framework may provide all students, including those with ASD, with the necessary level of support to ensure an effective educational environment." They also stated that currently students with an ASD are not having their individual needs met in mainstream classrooms. Best practice in educational settings when including students with an ASD, would be to ensure that environments are structured to accommodate these students' sensory processing needs, through activities that are integrated into the curriculum or daily activities (Baranek, 2002; Smith Roley et al., 2009). A whole group instruction approach prevents isolation and builds positive peer relationships (Smith et al. 2009). Kuypers (2013, p. 2), completed a case study using the 18 lesson program "The Zones of Regulation", which was based on self-regulation and sensory integration strategies, suggested that "it became apparent that the curriculum could reach a much broader population, due to the program being developed for students with disabilities."

Sensory Integration in Today's Classroom

Currently, there is no data available to show how sensory integration is used in the classroom on a whole or individual basis. Most research into sensory interventions is focused on the individual child, therefore, one can assume that the individual (exclusive) sensory integration strategies are the majority of classroom sensory interventions. The program being used in some mainstream and special educational settings today is called "*How does your engine run?: The Alert Program for Self-Regulation*" (Williams and Shellenberger, 1994). This program is a sensory-based approach that focuses on how a student's "engine is running", or how they are managing with their learning. The program uses a sensor motor approach and activities based on sensory integration theory. The 12-lesson program is designed to teach children to recognize when they need extra sensory input to stay alert and calm. The program's effectiveness was tested by Zielder (2012) over a six-week period with 7-10 year old students that displayed sensory processing difficulties: it was therefore not a whole class program. Nevertheless, the results were positive and teachers reported that students who received the intervention had improved attention when on-task, with the added bonus of increased communication between students, parents and teachers.

Roberts et al. (2007) concluded that sensory integration therapy in a clinical setting improved students' behaviour regulation within the classroom. They suggested that future research was needed to support the benefits of sensory integration therapy where the focus was on behavioral and learning outcomes, with comprehensive educational criteria, as did Baranek (2002, p. 417), after she revised and summarized 13 sensory integration based projects. Baranek (2002, p. 417) further suggested that large-scale educational models of sensory integration would be beneficial to further support current literature. Rogers (1998, cited Baranek 2002, pg. 417) summarized in her comprehensive review of educational programs, that the lack of data did not deem the intervention as ineffective, but that "efficacy has not been objectively demonstrated."

"Cool, Calm and Collected and Ready to Learn"

A whole class sensory regulation program called the "*Cool Calm Collected and Ready to Learn*" program (Collyer, 2014) may provide positive outcomes for students with sensory processing difficulties in education classrooms (Collyer, 2014, pg. 2) The aim of the "*Cool Calm Collected and Ready to Learn*" program builds upon current research in determining whether educational, curriculum and social goals are inhibited or facilitated with the implantation of an inclusive sensory regulation program.

The program is designed to be used a complementary intervention to further support the array of learning strategies already in place (Howe et al., 2004). Individual needs are responded to but articulated in an inclusive structure that does not exclude any student with sensory needs. The program is based on the idea of a Sensory diet (Wilbarger, 1995) and will focus on the three fundamental sensory systems: Proprioceptive, Vestibular and Tactile. Targeted activities that focus on the organisation of these fundamental systems will be used. The program will provide a controlled sensory input of these systems similar to Ayres (1979) Sensory Integration Theory. The aim of the program is to support students learning by regulating them into calm and alert states ready for learning.

The Sensory Profile School Companion (Dunn, 2006) can be used as tool to group together students who require the same type of sensory intervention to achieve a focused and ready to learn state. This will ensure that all activities in a sensory diet are individually focused and responsive. The program will link to all curriculum Key Learning Area's (KLA). Including links to the curriculum, and all students will benefit from participation in the inclusive sensory regulation program.

The program hypothesis is that all students will benefit in the regulation of the sensory systems that affect their ability to further engage in the classroom environment. The "*Cool Calm Collect and Ready to Learn*" program will be used as an essential tool throughout the day for regulation and learning readiness.

It will be designed to meet the needs of Early Stage One and Stage one (Kindergarten, Year one and Year two), as this age group is the fundamental age for building positive experiences with learning, school, social interactions and the basis for learning strategies for self-regulation (Deiner, 1993; Humphrey 2002).

Conclusion

Despite the mixed arguments surrounding the benefits of sensory regulation strategies, the growing body of research indicates that sensory regulation strategies has positive effects upon students with a sensory dysfunction. Baranek (2002, p. 406) summarizes his findings by stating "through sensory and vestibular activities actively controlled/sought out by the child, the nervous system is thought to be able to better modulate, organise, and integrate information from the environment, which in turn provides a foundation for further adaptive responses and higher-order learning." This is the overall goal of providing an inclusive sensory regulation program for students in an educational setting. As Ayres (1979) suggested, even "normal" children can have problems with sensory processing at one time or another, therefore the "*Cool Calm Collected and Ready to Learn*" sensory regulation program may provide many learning supports for all students in the education classroom. Larger scale, long term and statistical studies are needed to further understand the educational and classroom benefits of such intervention (Mailloux and Smith Roley, 2010).

References

Ayres, A. (1972). *Sensory Integration and Learning Disorders.* Western Psychological Services, Los Angeles.

Ayres, A. (1979). *Sensory Integration and the child, Western Psychological Services*, Los Angeles.

Ahn, R., Miller, L., Milberger, S., and McIntosh, D. (2004). "Prevalence of parents" perception of sensory processing disorders among kindergarten children" In: *American Journal of Occupational Therapy*, 58, 287-293.

Baranek, G. (2002). "Efficacy of sensory and motor interventions for children with Autism" in the *Journal of Autism and Developmental Disorders*, 32, 5, 397-422.

Biel, L. and Peske, N. (2009). *Raising a Sensory Smart Child*, Penguin Books Ltd. London, England.

Bodrova, E. and Leong, D. (2007). *Tools of the mind: The Vygotskian approach to early childhood education* (2nd ed.). Columbus, OH: Merrill/Prentice Hall.

Bundy, A., Lane, S. and Murray, E. (2002). *Sensory Integration: Theory and Practice*, 2nd Ed. F. Davies Publications.

Case-Smith, J. (2010). "Evidence-based Practice in Occupational Therapy for Children with an Autism Spectrum Disorder" In: *Autism: Comprehensive Occupational Therapy Approach*, Ed. Miller Kuhaneck and Watling. Chapter 23, American Occupational Therapy Association, Inc., 701-742.

Chandler-Olcott, K. and Kluth, P. (2009). "Why everyone benefits from including students with Autism in Literacy classrooms" In: *The Reading Teacher*, 62, 7, 548-557.

Cohn, E. (2000). "Parent perspectives of Occupational therapy using a sensory integration approach" In: *The American Journal of Occupation Therapy*, 55, 285-294.

Collyer, K. (2014). *Cool Calm Collected and ready to learn – a sensory regulation program for the infants' classroom.* University of New England, Armidale, Australia.

Culp, S., (2011). *A Buffet of Sensory Sensations*, AAPP Publishing, Kansas, US.

Deiner, P. L., (1993), *Resources for teaching children with diverse abilities,* 2nd edn. Harcourt Brace and Company.

Devlin, S., Healy, O., Leader, G., and Hughes, B. (2010). "Comparison of behavior intervention and sensory-integration therapy in the treatment of Challenging behavior" In: *Journal of Autism and Developmental Disorders*, 41, 1303-1320.

Dunn, W. (1997). "The impacts of sensory processing abilities on the daily lives of young children and their families: a conceptual model" In: *Infants and Young Children*, 9, 4, 23-35.

Dunn, W. (1999). *The Sensory Profile*, Psychological Corporation, Texas.

Dunn, W. (2001). "The sensations of everyday life: Empirical, theoretical, and pragmatic considerations" In: *American Journal of Occupational Therapy*, 55, 608-620.

Dunn, W. (2006). *The sensory profile school companion.* San Antonio, TX. Psychological Corporation.

Dunn, W. and Donaldson, C. (2001) "Integration of the sensorimotor approach in the classroom" In: *A sensorimotor approach to management*, Chapter 12, Aspen Publishers, Inc. Gaithersburg, Maryland, 297-311.

Dunn, W., Saiter, J. and Rinner, L. (2002). "Asperger Syndrome and sensory processing" In: *Focus on Autism and Other Developmental Disabilities*, 17, 3, 172-185.

Frederickson, N., Jones, A. and Lang, J. (2010). "Inclusive provision options for pupils on the autistic spectrum" In: *Journal of Research in Special Educational Needs*, 10, 2, 63-73.

Glennon, T. 2010. "An introduction to the Autism Spectrum Disorders" In: *Autism: Comprehensive Occupational Therapy Approach*, Ed. Miller Kuhaneck and Watling. Chapter 1, American Occupational Therapy Association, Inc., 3-24.

Gourley, L., Wind, C., Henninger, E. M., and Chinitz, S. (2012). "Sensory processing difficulties, behavioral problems, and parental stress in a clinical population of young children" In: *Journal of Family Studies*, 22. 912-921.

Grandin, T. (1995). *Thinking in Pictures.* Vintage Publications, US.

Grey, I., Bruton, C., Honan, R., McGuinness, R., and Daly, M. (2007). "Co-operative learning for children with Autistic Spectrum Disorder (ASD) in Mainstream and Special Class settings: An exploratory study", In: *Educational Psychology in Practice: Theory, research and practice in education psychology*, 23, 4, 317-327.

Howe, M., Brittain, L. and McCathren, R. (2004). "Meeting the sensory needs of young children in classrooms" In: *Young Exceptional Children*, 8, 1, 11-19.

Huebner, R. (Ed), (2001). *Autism: A sensorimotor approach to management*, Aspen Publishers, Inc. Gaithersburg, Maryland.

Huebner, R. and Dunn, W. (2001). "Introduction and Basic Concepts" In: *A sensorimotor approach to management*, Chapter 1, pp. 3-37. Aspen Publishers, Inc. Gaithersburg, Maryland.

Humphrey, R. (2002). "Young children's occupations: explicating the dynamics of developmental processes" In: *American Journal of Occupational Therapy*, 56, 171-179.

Humphrey, N. and Lewis, S. (2008). "What does inclusion mean for pupils on the Autistic spectrum in mainstream secondary schools?" In: *Journal of Research in Special Education Needs*, 8, 3, 132-140.

Kientz, M. and Dunn, W. (1997). "A comparison of the performance of children with and without autism on the sensory profile" In: *The American Journal of Occupational Therapy*, 51, 530-537.

Kuypers. L. (2013). "Sensory integration", In: *American Occupational Therapy Association*, Inc. 36, 4.

Leblanc, L., Richardson, W. and Burns, K. (2009). "Autism spectrum disorder and the inclusive classroom", In: *Teacher education and special education: the Journal of Teacher Education division of the Council for Exceptional Children*, 32, 2, 166-179.

Lynch, S. and Irvine, A. (2009). "Inclusive education and best practice for children with Autism Spectrum Disorder: An Integrated Approach", In: *International Journal of Inclusive Education*, 13, 8, 845-859.

Mailloux, Z. and Smith Roley, S. (2010). "Sensory integration" In: *Autism: Comprehensive Occupational Therapy Approach*, Ed. Miller Kuhaneck and Watling. Chapter 17, American Occupational Therapy Association, Inc. 469-508.

McIntosh, D., Ahn, R. Miller, L. J., and Milberger, S. (1999). "Prevalence of Parents' Perceptions of Sensory Processing Disorders Among Kindergarten Children", *The American Journal of Occupational Therapy*, 58, 3, 287-293.

Murray-Slutsky, C. and Paris, B. 2000, *Exploring the Spectrum of Autism and Pervasive Developmental Disorders: Intervention strategies, The Therapy skill builders*, Harcourt Health Sciences Company, US.

Oetter, P., Richter, E. W. and Frick, S. 1993. *MORE integrating the mouth with sensory and postural functions*. Hugo, MN: PDP Press.

O'Neill, M. and Jones, R. (1997). "Sensory Perceptual Abnormalities in Autism: A case for research?", In: *Journal of Autism and Developmental Disabilities*, 27, 283-293.

Parham, L. and Mailloux, Z. (2005). "Sensory Integration" In: *Occupational Therapy for Children*, Case-Smith (Ed.), 5th Edn. St Louis, Moseby.

Prudhomme White, B., Mulligan, S., Merril, K., and Wright, J. (2007). "An examination of the relationships between motor and process kills and scores on the sensory profile" In: *American Journal of Occupational Therapy*, 61, 2, 154-160.

Roberts, J., King-Thomas, L. and Boccia, M. (2007). "Behavioral indexes of efficacy of sensory integration therapy" In: *The American Journal of Occupational Therapy*, 61, 5, 555-563.

Schaff, R. and Miller, L. (2005). "Occupational therapy using a sensory integrative approach for children with developmental disabilities" In: *Mental Retardation and Developmental Research Reviews*, 11, 143-148.

Schaff, R. and Nightlinger, K. (2007). "Occupational therapy using a sensory integrative approach: a case study of effectiveness", In: *American Journal of Occupational Therapy*, 61, 239-246.

Smith Roley, S., Bissell, J. and Frolek Clark, G. 2009, "Providing Occupational Therapy Using Sensory Integration Theory and Methods in School-based Practice" In: *The American Journal of Occupational Therapy*, November/December (2009). 63, 6, 835-838.

Smith Myles, B., Tapscott Cook, K., Miller, N., Rinner, L., and Robbins, L. (2001). *Asperger Syndrome and Sensory issues.* Autism Publishing Co. Shawnee Mission, Kansas.

Vargas, S. and Camilli, G. (1999). "A meta-analysis of research on sensory integration treatment" In: *American Journal of Occupational Therapy,* 53, 2, 189-198.

Watling, R., Henry, D. and Miller-Kuhaneck, H. (2006). "Sensory integration: its not just for children" In: *American Occupational Therapy Association* Inc., 29, 4, 1-3.

Watling, R., Davies, P., Patten Koenig, K., and Scaff, R. (2011). *Occupational Therapy Practice Guidelines for Children and Adolescents with Challenges in Sensory processing and Sensory integration*, American Occupational Therapy Association, Inc. US.

Wilbarger, P. (1995). "The sensory diet: activity programs based on sensory processing theory" In: *Sensory Integration Special Interest Section Newsletter*, 18, 2.

Wilkinson, L. (2007). "Supporting the inclusion of a student with Asperger Syndrome: A case study using conjoint behavioral consultation and self management" In: *Educational Psychology in Practice: Theory, Research and Practice in Educational Psychology,* 21, 4, 307-326.

Williams, M. and Shellenberger, S. (1994). *How does your engine run: the alert program for self-regulation.* Therapy Words, New Mexico, US.

Wilson, B., Kaplan, B., Fellowes, S., Grunchy, C., and Faris, P. (1992) "The efficacy of sensory integration treatment compared to tutoring" In: *Physical and Occupational therapy in Paediatrics*, 12, 1, 1-36.

Yack, E., Aquilla, P. and Sutton, S. (2002). *Building Bridges through sensory integration*, 2nd Ed. Sensory Resources, US.

Zeilder, S. (2012). "Sensory Processing Challenges in the Schools" In: *OT Practice*, June 4, 2012, 14-19.

In: Asperger Syndrome
Editor: Michael F. Shaughnessy
ISBN: 978-1-63463-810-4

Chapter 3

Management Strategies for Students with Asperger's

Effie Laman*[*] *and Leigh Kackley-Smith
Texas Tech University, TX, US

Abstract

When attempting to design a program for someone who has a different perspective and interpretation of life, it is essential to empathise with their position. Children with Asperger's Syndrome typically exhibit social awkwardness and an all-absorbing interest in specific topics. In this chapter we will look at the management strategies and coordination of services needed to be in place for the student with AS for students from birth to college.

Keywords: Asperger Syndrome, management, coordination

Introduction

The manifestation of Asperger Syndrome is unique for each individual and family. While most "Aspie's" share significant social disability, many are very successful academically while others struggle to simply accomplish some type of meaningful work. Individuals with AS may have an intense intellectual interest in a specific area of study; others may become fixated on a topic that seems to be of no practical use. Some "Aspie's" may maintain a few friendships, others are desperately lonely. Therefore, each student with AS has specific educational needs that will require an individualized educational program.

However, the special education road is complicated and laborious resulting in a long, difficult, and often scary path that families must navigate as they begin the process of diagnostic screening and assessment while trying to find answers to their questions and

[*] Corresponding author: Email: Mrs.laman@hotmail.com.

concerns regarding their child. From the initial suspicion of AS to diagnosis, to educational planning – there will be a need for collaboration between families and the professionals that will be providing services to their child. This chapter will provide an overview of research regarding how best to help families manage this team of service providers as they embark on this journey called special education.

The Special Education Process

Lawson and Sailor (2000) distilled the Special Education process into 10 basic steps.

Step 1. Child is identified as possibly needing special education and related services.

There are two primary ways in which children are identified as possibly needing special education and related services: the system known as *Child Find* (which operates in each state), and by referral of a parent or school personnel. Each state is required by IDEA to identify, locate, and evaluate all children with disabilities in the state who need special education and related services. To do so, states conduct what are known as Child Find activities. When a child is identified by Child Find as possibly having a disability and as needing special education, parents may be asked for permission to evaluate their child. Parents can also call the Child Find office and ask that their child be evaluated. A school professional may ask that a child be evaluated to see if he or she has a disability. Parents may also contact the child's teacher or other school professional to ask that their child be evaluated. This request may be verbal, but it's best to put it in writing. Parental consent is needed before a child may be evaluated. Under the federal IDEA regulations, evaluation needs to be completed within 60 days after the parent gives consent. However, if a State's IDEA regulations give a different timeline for completion of the evaluation, the State's timeline is applied.

Step 2. Child is evaluated.

Evaluation is an essential early step in the special education process for a child. It's intended to answer these questions:

- Does the child have a disability that requires the provision of special education and related services?
- What are the child's specific educational needs?
- What special education services and related services, then, are appropriate for addressing those needs?

By law, the initial evaluation of the child must be "full and individual"— focused on that child and that child alone. The evaluation must assess the child in all areas related to the child's suspected disability. The evaluation results will be used to decide the child's eligibility for special education and related services and to make decisions about an appropriate educational program for the child. If the parents disagree with the evaluation, they have the right to take their child for an Independent Educational Evaluation (IEE). They can ask that the school system pay for this IEE.

Step 3. Eligibility is decided.

A group of qualified professionals and the parents look at the child's evaluation results. Together, they decide if the child is a "child with a disability," as defined by IDEA. If the parents do not agree with the eligibility decision, they may ask for a hearing to challenge the decision.

Step 4. Child is found eligible for services.

If the child is found to be a child with a disability, as defined by IDEA, he or she is eligible for special education and related services. Within 30 calendar days after a child is determined eligible, a team of school professionals and the parents must meet to write an individualized education program (IEP) for the child.

Step 5. IEP meeting is scheduled.

The school system schedules and conducts the IEP meeting. School staff must:

- contact the participants, including the parents;
- notify parents early enough to make sure they have an opportunity to attend;
- schedule the meeting at a time and place agreeable to parents and the school;
- tell the parents the purpose, time, and location of the meeting;
- tell the parents who will be attending; and
- tell the parents that they may invite people to the meeting who have knowledge or special expertise about the child.

Step 6. IEP meeting is held and the IEP is written.

The IEP team gathers to talk about the child's needs and write the student's IEP. Parents and the student (when appropriate) are full participating members of the team. If the child's placement (where the child will receive his or her special education and related services) is decided by a different group, the parents must be part of that group as well.

Before the school system may provide special education and related services to the child for the first time, the parents must give consent. The child begins to receive services as soon as possible after the IEP is written and this consent is given. If the parents do not agree with the IEP and placement, they may discuss their concerns with other members of the IEP team and try to work out an agreement. If they still disagree, parents can ask for mediation, or the school may offer mediation. Parents may file a state complaint with the state education agency or a due process complaint, which is the first step in requesting a due process hearing, at which time mediation must be available.

Step 7. After the IEP is written, services are provided.

The school makes sure that the child's IEP is carried out as it was written. Parents are given a copy of the IEP. Each of the child's teachers and service providers has access to the IEP and knows his or her specific responsibilities for carrying out the IEP. This includes the accommodations, modifications, and supports that must be provided to the child, in keeping with the IEP.

Step 8. Progress is measured and reported to parents.

The child's progress toward the annual goals as stated in the IEP are measured. Parents are regularly informed of their child's progress and whether that progress is sufficient for the child to achieve stated goals by the end of the year. These progress reports must be given to parents at least as often as parents are informed of their nondisabled children's progress.

Step 9. IEP is reviewed.

The child's IEP is reviewed by the IEP team at least once a year, or more often if the parents or school ask for a review. If necessary, the IEP is revised. Parents, as team members, must be invited to participate in these meetings. Parents can make suggestions for changes, can agree or disagree with the IEP, and agree or disagree with the placement. If parents do not agree with the IEP and placement, they may discuss their concerns with other members of the IEP team and try to work out an agreement. There are several options, including additional testing, an independent evaluation, or asking for mediation, or a due process hearing. They may also file a complaint with the state education agency.

Step 10. Child is reevaluated.

The child must be reevaluated at least every three years. This evaluation is sometimes called a "triennial" and serves to determine if the child still has a disability as defined by IDEA, and if so, the educational needs of the child. However, the child must be reevaluated more often if conditions warrant or if the child's parent or teacher asks for a new evaluation.

As demonstrated by the above list, many professionals will come and go in the life of a child with a diagnosis of AS and therefore, their family. This management team composed of the child (when able), parents and family members, and professional service providers is vital for the individual with Asperger's successful achievement. Australian researchers, Prior and Roberts (2012) found that families with children that have autism should be meaningfully involved in their child's management in special education from the beginning assessment through program development and implementation of services, until their child with autism is mature enough to meaningfully advocate for self.

The Management Team

Management is the coordination of the collaborative teams formed for the express purpose of helping the child with AS to achieve success and is a process of stages including forming, storming, norming, performing, and adjourning (Tuckman & Jensen, 1977). Management teams may be needed for short periods of time, but due to the nature of Asperger Syndrome, the team may need to stay in place throughout the lifespan of the individual with AS. However, the members of the team may need to change as the child transitions from one developmental stage to the next. Parents are in a position to offer continuity to the transition process and should be groomed to be the leader of their child's management (collaborative) team.

The management team should be sensitive to the stresses encountered by families of children with autism, especially during times of their child's transition from one life stage to the next. There are many great resources for each stage of transition. The parent has many choices for resources and should be open to the local or State Autism recommendations. The Lawrence (2013) text, *Finding Asperger Syndrome in the Family: A Book of Answers* is an excellent resource that provides parents of children with Asperger Syndrome with practical advice on how to prepare their child for moving to a new school and how to help make the transition as smooth as possible. A wide range of material is covered, including useful guidance on choosing the right school, supporting the child during the period prior to the move, and identifying and practicing the different social rules and expectations of the new school. Strategies covered in the book include working out a transition time-line, identifying a named adult and "safe haven" at the school, and effective communication between parents, teachers and support staff.

Parent Involvement

Research indicates that the earlier parents become involved in their child's educational process, the more powerful the effects will be. Educators frequently point out the critical role of the home and family environment in determining children's school success, and it appears that the earlier this influence is "harnessed," the greater the likelihood of higher student achievement. Early childhood education programs with strong parental involvement components have amply demonstrated the effectiveness of this approach. Participants in Barnhill's (2003) research largely attributed their ability to persevere in college to decisions they had made with their parents. Barnhill (2014) found that the impact of parental involvement and active participation in formal transition planning is such that it is imperative that the family become expert managers of their child's educational program. There are literally hundreds of books, journal articles, and stand-alone reports regarding parents' involvement in their children's education including research, expert opinions, theory papers, program descriptions, and guidelines for setting up programs. A great many of these reports are informative and useful, and, because parent involvement has become a "hot topic" in the past few years, there is considerable current information (Family, 2012).

Each child with Asperger's is an individual with unique needs. Therefore, each family situation will require specific interventions. A few more global suggestions that may be useful for parents and families are provided here:

- Keep the environment predictable and familiar, and prepare your child for changes. For example count down the time until a transition.
- Prime your child for new situations by explaining in advance what you expect will happen, and prepare them for the "what if's." For example, explain you are going to visit grandpa, but "what if" grandpa doesn't answer the door.
- Provide consistent structure and routine.
- Many children respond well to visual supports, such as a daily schedule using pictures. Schedules help to give information about what is happening during the day and give a place for the child to check when needed (just like you might check your planner or shopping list).
- Pay attention to sensory input from the environment, like noise, temperature, smells, crowds, etc. (Coucouvanis & Boyse, 2014).

Public School

Families may need help making an honest appraisal of the specific strengths and challenges their children face and in determining if the student's school is willing and able to address these needs. We know from experience that children with Asperger Syndrome cannot develop these skills on their own. The earlier that appropriate interventions are in place the more likely it is that their independence potential is maximized and positive outcomes will be achieved. Possible school solutions include:

1. Engaging a consultant to educate the student's school and help with specific intervention strategies.
2. Hiring a trained paraprofessional to work with the student.
3. Providing support services when needed such as speech and language therapy, occupational therapy, physical therapy, and counseling.
4. Finding a special education school capable of providing the level of academic support and challenge needed.
5. Placing the child in a specialized setting for students with Asperger Syndrome that addresses all of the above while providing a peer group and self-advocacy model.

A professional familiar with the wide array of characteristics of AS can help families make a professional assessment of a child's real needs and how they are currently being addressed. Each stage of development brings new challenges to children and families. The management team must be cognizant of the need to match the student's strengths and needs with the current academic situation. A school that was able to provide a wonderful environment in third grade may not be able to address the new challenges that middle school brings. Therefore, an objective reappraisal of the student's maturity and the appropriateness of the educational situation is a critical part of academic and personal success from preschool through college.

"Least restrictive placement" is an educational term that means that students should be provided with the proper level of support for success without placing them in unnecessarily restrictive environments. For students with Asperger Syndrome, the level of support that is necessary to help them optimize their skills and strengths without removing them from typical school experiences should be provided. Some students may need a protective environment, some may need learning supports, while others may need a little support developing their social skills in a regular education setting. Matching the individual need to the level of support is critical to helping a child gain self-esteem and independence.

Families should consider how the following potential difficulties are being addressed in the school setting.

1. The development of basic social skills and social relationship abilities. School programs and community clinicians often provide social skills training. The quality and type of this training, however, is critical to progress. Many activities called social skills are not based in solid research. Just because someone provides a child with opportunities for social interaction does not make the activity a useful social skills development experience. Specific skills at the child's level of need

coupled with opportunities for generalization outside of the formal training situation are necessary components for skill development to occur. Children with Asperger Syndrome typically have had great difficulty acquiring skills that typical children simply pick up from their environment. Those with AS need specific help to perceive, acquire, and generalize basic social skills. Parents should always ask social skills trainers if they are utilizing proven, evidence-based techniques. If parents are not involved in the program, a vital link for generalizability is lost and families should be somewhat suspect of the program. Sometimes social skills programs are too simplistic, teaching only the basic instrumental skills such as eye contact and greeting. Helping individuals understand social norms and develop more sophisticated social cognition skills are critical for relationship development.

Although a parent may be overjoyed that there is any social skills opportunity, it is still necessary to be a critical consumer and request a detailed statement of philosophy and curriculum, whether it is a school or a private practitioner in the community. If basic social skills have been acquired, children with Asperger Syndrome may continue to experience difficulty developing authentic relationships. Their interests may be atypical or age inappropriate or they may have all their social overtures rejected by others. Teachers and related service providers can facilitate interactions in the real life situations that school provides, particularly on the playground, at lunch, and in other unstructured situations.

Parents often ask what to do when their children are unable to make friends. Parents can help their children find others with shared interests. Finding another who loves Warhammer, entomology, or chess goes a long way toward starting a relationship. Parents and teachers can be creative in finding appropriate peers with similar interests through clubs, internet sites, or other personal resources. Putting random children together who share only the diagnosis of AS (and consequently poorly developed social skills) is far less effective than finding two children who are both fascinated by the same activity and can talk endlessly about it together. Even when an appropriate peer has been found, and the children seem to be a good match, adults should bear in mind that their facilitation of social interaction can help immensely, especially in the early stages of acquaintanceship.

2. Organizational problems within the context of good academic skills. Problems with disorganization are very common for students with AS and frequently have a negative impact on achievement. If a child has these problems, asking him to be more organized or providing negative consequences are ineffective and painful interventions. A neuropsychological evaluation can help us understand exactly what underlying skill deficits are causing these students to lose their initial academic advantage. A student who processes information more slowly than others, or who can't set priorities, or who doesn't understand the passage of time, or who over focuses on details and never finishes work (and these are all fairly typical of individuals with AS) will have less and less success with academics over time and lose that important source of self-esteem. If the underlying problems are identified and specified on an IEP, finding a way to support the student's organizational difficulties becomes an educational imperative, rather than a source of personal criticism. For an unclassified student, the specific recommendations of a neuropsychological evaluation can lead to more specified help and a less likely

tendency to blame rather than support. Parents should be ready to suggest a consultant who can educate teachers and other school staff in fundamental brain differences and how they manifest in this population as many educators do not know this important information.

3. Immature or inappropriate emotional expression.
   A fairly common result of having limited friendships is that emotional maturity is slow to develop and sometimes develops in an odd way, causing daily social pain. Emotional regulation is a developmental skill that arises as an interaction between one's basic brain mechanisms and the daily experiences with others. Children with AS often have differences in the neural circuitry responsible for emotional development. These differences may color their experiences in the world. Furthermore, through self-isolation, limited numbers of relationships or peer rejection, the opportunity for social-emotional learning may be less than for typical children. These difficulties play out in school as immature social regulation, inability to modulate response to disappointment or frustration, or anger in response to any deviation from expectancy. Immature behavior further distances the student with AS from others, and may jeopardize the school placement. School personnel often have not been trained in specific techniques to support children having these problems. A behavior plan that is too simple tends to exacerbate rather than help a child who is losing emotional control because of complex brain related issues. A consultant, who is highly experienced in the emotional development of children and adolescents with AS, can be invaluable in helping a school develop a protocol to manage and support this kind of student. This may help a child maintain school placement and contribute to the development of more socially appropriate emotional regulation.
4. Isolation, anxiety, and depression.
   Often children with Asperger Syndrome retreat to the internet or a fantasy world to avoid social anguish. Families are often at a loss as to how to change these behaviors. Sometimes schools are punitive when students cannot attend, blaming the student for being manipulative or the parents for not exerting discipline. Students with AS who are showing excessive isolation should be evaluated for an anxiety or mood disorder. Changes from baseline functioning, such as an increase in irritability or aggression should also be evaluated from a mental health perspective. Anxiety or mood disorders are treatable problems that require close cooperation between the school and the family. Schools can help by investigating sources of fear or anxiety that the child with AS may exhibit, they can help families find appropriate professionals that can assist with these types of behavior, and they can cooperate with families in treatment protocols. Families should take potential anxiety and depression seriously, not view these issues as an inevitable part of AS, and seek appropriate treatment.
5. Wide variations in development.
   Students with AS characteristically exhibit wide disparities in basic abilities. Typical difficulties directly attributable to brain function include poor coordination, handwriting difficulties, slow processing, inattention, and extremes in academic ability. It is more difficult to be a person with widely varying abilities because expectancies are often unrealistic. Just because a student can solve arithmetic problems mentally does not mean that the student can keep order in long division. Just because a student can speak with erudition about history does not mean that

writing mature compositions about history is possible. It is critical to understand strengths and weaknesses so that weaknesses can be identified and supported and, just as importantly, intellect can be challenged. Sometimes language or motor function can sabotage other skill areas. Consequently, even for older students, regular Speech and Language, Occupational Therapy, and Physical Therapy evaluations are critical to address unevenness of academic performance and to help develop important interventions to support ongoing academic progress.

As the child with AS transitions from one developmental stage to the next and the educational program shifts focus, trust becomes a central issue as some members of the management team may leave while others are added. Each team member will bring a different perspective, experience, knowledge, and skill set to the group. Based on their respective roles - parents, family members, and educators are trusted to independently analyze and respond to situations in a way that has the child's best interests at heart. Such an attitude supports the notion that collaboratively achieved solutions will, in the majority of cases, best meet students' and families' needs. According to Fiedler, Simpson, & Clark (2007) such a process necessitates professionals and family members to be sensitive to the perceptions and perspectives of others, and be willing to attempt to understand their frame of reference. Such a process promotes a collaborative, solution-oriented problem-solving process that is characterized by openness to a number of possible solutions to problems that arise in the course of meeting of students' and families need.

Each member of the management team should be an advocate for the individual child as they share the responsibility of reducing barriers and creating an environment for the child's success as charged by IDEA 2004 and NCLB Acts. Such collaboration is, by its very nature, team-driven and multidisciplinary, with communication being the cornerstone. Strategies for good collaborative teams, and barriers to overcome in communication, are addressed in the following section.

Communication

Collaboration tends to steer both professionals and family members. Wahlberg (2002) prompts the manager and team to understand that stress in the individual with AS and family members are multiplied times 10. New routines, new requirements, and new patterns can be very challenging for someone with AS. The management team's ultimate goal is to prepare an educational plan that will ensure that programs and transitions provide adequate time for the individual with AS and their family to acclimate and adjust to each new stage of development (Wahlberg, 2012). Not surprisingly, the importance of effective communication in furthering parent and family support has been prominently noted for decades. For instance, Dewey (1938) suggested that listening is a key element of effective communication and a significant vehicle for facilitating feelings of acceptance and value in others. Dale Carnegie (1936) similarly noted that effective communication involves, by its very nature, demonstrating interest in another person, and thus is a basic means of establishing rapport. Although often overlooked because of its ubiquitous nature and perceived simplicity, use of effective communication methods is an essential and foundational emotional and psychological tool (Fiedler, Simpson, & Clark, 2007).

Six Strategies to Improve Communication and Collaboration

The strategies are built on Kochhar-Bryant (2007) model on how to improve communication and collaboration with emphasis on team building for students with Asperger's.

Strategy 1. Affirm the importance of the child and the common goal of the collaboration for the child's success.

Strategy 2. Build a personal commitment to the child and the collaborative process.

Strategy 3. Build a common commitment to the power of the team. Create an appreciation for and commitment of each member.

Strategy 4. Clearly communicate the rules of engagement to establish a climate for constructive collaboration.

All collaborators must feel safe in the group process and feel that their expertise and experience is valued and respected. The expected outcomes of this strategy include a team process that is characterized by (a) constructive dialog; (b) respect for diverse opinions; (c) a reflective approach to conflict, moving beyond impulsive or defensive reactions, and toward deeper interpretation of conflicts and concerns in terms of the over goal; and (d) a set of governing principles that shape team behavior, help troubleshoot threats to collaboration along the way, and serve as the basis for team performance.

Strategy 5. Facilitate the sharing of knowledge, new information, and prior experience.

Strategy 6. Address problematic behavior swiftly and constructively. The manager or team leader must remain aware that sometimes individual behaviors can undermine and threaten the work of and survival of the team.

Ten Blocks to Effective Communication and Strategies to Overcome Them

Communication habits of team members may undermine the efforts of the group diverting the group from their purpose of providing the best educational plan for the child with AS. Peter Gerlach (2003), professional trauma-recovery and family systems therapist, presented habits and behaviors that can block communication between group members and offered solutions. Adapted from his Gerlach's (2003) work these are some of the barriers and solutions:

1. *Unequal Status.* Someone in the team sends a verbal or nonverbal message (unconscious message sent through voice or body language) that is received as "*I*

don't view you or respect you as an equal on this team." The manger should be aware that communication is effective only when each participant believes that they have equal status with others and feel respected.

2. *Mismatch in Communication.* Two or more team members' communication needs conflict—for example, the parent needs to "vent" or express frustration, and the diagnostician needs to persuade the parent to adopt an idea. The communications are mismatched and can create conflicts, which could be avoided if team members are aware of each other's need for information or need for time to digest the information, and understand that different needs can conflict at times.
3. *Mixed Message.* A team member may communicate a double or mixed message (their words say one thing and their voice or manner imply another (e.g., the person shouts—"*I am NOT angry with you*" with arms folded tightly across the chest). The response to such communication is often confusion and distrust of the person speaking. Such double messages occur when the speaker has two conflicting thoughts at the same time and is not honest in his or her communication. The team can help the speaker to become aware of the double message being sent.
4. *Distraction.* One or more team members are distracted in the team meeting and can't focus or attend well to the work of the group. They may be distracted by (a) physical discomfort (e.g., pain, thirst, sleepiness, full bladders, headaches); (b) worry, anxiety, or other strong emotion; or (c) environmental factors such as noise, sirens, flashing lights, or room temperature, and yet they try to communicate in the group. The manager should be aware of the potential for environmental and personal distractions.
5. *Interruptions.* When a team member frequently interrupts the group, they are communicating an implicit message "*I'm superior and my needs and ideas are more important than yours.*" This behavior also suggest that the interrupting team member is preparing his or her response without really listening to the other, or is rushing the speaker. The other person may feel discounted or insulted and may react with defensiveness or resentment. The most constructive response in a team situation is to respectfully make the interrupter aware of the behavior and calmly say, "*I really need you to stop interrupting me.*"
6. *Withholding Emotions.* Sometimes people withhold emotions either purposefully or unconsciously as they communicate. Others in the group are left feeling unsafe or confused about the person's meaning or may misinterpret them (*You don't trust me because you are hiding something*). Chronic anxiety and distrust in the group can result. However, some people (particularly the "harm avoiders") have difficulty expressing emotions and need encouragement to understand how this communication block hinders effective problem solving and creativity.
7. *Focus on the Past.* Occasionally a team member may have the habit of focusing continually on the past or the future "We've tried that in the past and it didn't work"; "I know what's going to happen in the future, so your suggestion isn't going to work"). Such behavior can be deliberate or unconscious, but usually serves to avoid confronting problems in the present. The team member needs an awareness of how this behavior affects communication effectiveness and relationships. The team member is also seeking reassurance that patterns of the past will not be repeated.

8. *Focus on Self.* Some individuals are habitually self-centered, causing others to feel ignored or resentful. They may repeatedly or suddenly change the subject to divert the conversation, or they may exhibit nonstop talking which undermines communication and keeps people at an emotional distance. Awareness and respectful assertion on the part of the other team members can intervene constructively ("*I notice that you change the subject when we talk about the program*").
9. *Preaching or Moralizing.* A team member may have the habit of preaching to others or advising them, which can undermine team relationships, implying—"*I know how to fix your problem and you don't.*" If someone needs to express their feelings or to vent, they want to be respectfully heard and don't necessarily need to have someone insist on "fixing" the problem.
10. *Withdrawal and Lack of Eye Contact.* Physical or emotional withdrawal can communicate to others: "*You scare or overwhelm me*," or "*I am not interested in what you have to say right now*." Habitual lack of eye contact can also communicate to others a feeling of inferiority or intimidation which, over time, may result in loss of respect by team members and ineffective communication. Either message undermines communication and leaves others frustrated *("Greg, every time I suggest that we try a different approach in the classroom, you just say "fine" and then become silent. Is there something that's troubling you?).* Constructive communication involves honest feedback to the individual in order to respectfully explore what is triggering the withdrawal.

School and community professionals have a shared responsibility to assist parents and families in addressing their need for emotional and psychological support and identification of coping strategies (Lawson & Sailor, 2000). School personnel and school organizations play a primary as well as ongoing role in creating the foundation for emotional support (Fiedler, Simpson, & Clark, 2007). Through the development of collaborative relationships in which partners trust the intentions of the individual members of the group, effective information-exchange programs are created and parents and family members of individuals with AS are afforded the basic supports needed to function in the midst of AS related issues and challenges. According to Fiedler, Simpson, & Clark (2007) school personnel and school organizations do not typically have the resources and expertise to address the entire spectrum of parent and family emotional and psychological issues; therefore, community programs are need to provide these types of services. Administrators, teachers, and related service personnel - particularly school counselors, school social workers, and school psychologists, are encouraged to become more adept at referring parents and family members to appropriate community programs, personnel, agencies, and organizations for psychological counseling and other forms of clinical and social assistance (Bauer & Shea, 2003).

Conclusion

Professional collaboration has become more important in recent years as schools are being held accountable for the academic achievement of all students, including those with AS (Kochhar-Bryant, 2008). There is much research linking collaboration with student achievement. Professional-to-professional, teacher-to-student, special educator-to-general educator, and teacher-to-parent collaboration are all essential for effective case management (Abrams & Giggs, 2000; Attwood, 2007; Booth & Dunn, 2013, & Desimone, Smith, & Phillips, 2013). Collaboration among the IEP team members as well as school to community partnerships are vital to the successful achievement of individuals with AS (Dettmer, Dyke, & Thurson, 2005; Fiedler, Simpson, & Clark, 2007).

If the collaborative team is to remain in place for more than a short time, the human element takes on profound importance as the group seeks to work together to meet the educational needs of the student with AS. The success of the management team depends on effective interpersonal relationships and communication (Ohrt, Prochenko, Stulmaker, Huffman, Fernando, & Swan, 2014); the quality of the relationships between team members depend on the skills, beliefs, and attitudes of those involved (Kochhar-Bryant, 2007). Therefore, attention to and respect for the individual needs of each team member is necessary in order to create an environment in which the group functions effectively in making educational decisions for the individual with AS.

Families with children who have Asperger Syndrome must learn to navigate a long and arduous road as they begin the process of securing special education services for their child. A team approach has been found to be effective in empowering families as they seek to secure appropriate services for their child. School personnel, as well as professionals within the community, must come together to provide the appropriate programs and services for individuals with AS, and to come alongside families as they work to provide appropriate communication and social interaction, including effective behavior management for their child with AS (Garfinkle & Kaiser, 2004; Schertz & Odom, 2007; Tschirhart, Christensen, R., & Perry, J., 2005; van Garderen, Stormont, & Goel, 2012). In addition to increased achievement for individuals with AS, management teams provide much needed support and encouragement to families as they make this journey into the world of special education.

References

Abrams, L. S. & Gibbs, J. T. (2000). Planning for School Change School-Community Collaboration in a Full-Service Elementary School. *Urban Education, 35*(1), 79-103.

Attwood, T. (2007). *The complete guide to Asperser's syndrome.* London and Philadelphia: Jessica Kingsley Publishers.

Barnhill, G. P. (2014). Supporting Students With Asperger Syndrome on College Campuses Current Practices. *Focus on Autism and Other Developmental Disabilities*, 1088357614523121.

Bauer, A. M. & Shea, T. M. (2003). *Parents and schools: Creating a successful partnership for students with special needs*. Upper Saddle River, NM: Marrill Prentice Hall.

Booth, A. & Dunn, J. F. (Eds.). (2013). *Family-school links: How do they affect educational outcomes?* London: Routledge.

Carnegie, D. (1936). How to win friends and influence people. New York: Simon & Schuster.

Coucouvanis, J. & Boyse, K. (2014). Your child development & behavior resources: A guide to information and support for parents. University of Michigan Health System. Retrieved from http://www.med.umich.edu/yourchild/topics/autism.htm.

Desimone, L., Smith, T. & Phillips, K. (2013). Linking student achievement growth to professional development participation and changes in instruction: A longitudinal study of elementary students and teachers in Title I schools. *Teachers College Record*, *115*(5), 1-46.

Dettmer, P., Dyck, N. & Thurston, L. P. (2005). Consultation, collaboration, and teamwork for students with special needs.

Dewey, J. (1938). *Experience and education*. New York: Collier.

Family Resource Coalition of America. (2012). *How are we doing? A program self-assessment toolkit for the family support field*. Chicago: Author.

Fiedler, C. R., Simpson, R. L. & Clark, D. M. (2007). *Parents and Families of Children with Disabilities: Effective School-Based Support*. Pearson: Upper Saddle River, NJ.

Garfinkle, A. & Kaiser, A. P. (2004). Communication. In C. H. Kennedy & E. Horn (Eds.). *Including students with severe disabilities*. Boston: Allyn & Bacon.

Gerlach, P. K. (2003). *Satisfactions: 7 Relationship Skills You Need to Know*. Bloomington IN: Xlibris Corporation.

Kochhar-Brayant, C. A. (2008). Collaboration and system coordination for students with special needs: From early childhood to the postsecondary years. Pearson: Upper Saddle River, NJ.

Lawrence, C. (2013). *Finding Asperger Syndrome in the Family: A Book of Answers*. London: Straightforward co Ltd.

Lawson, H. A. & Sailor, W. (2000). Integrating services collaborating, and developing connenctions with schools. *Focus on Exceptional Children*, *33*(2), 1-22.

Prior, M. & Roberts, J. (2012). Early intervention for children with autism spectrum disorders: Guidelines for good practice' 2012. Retrieved from: *http://www.fahcsia.gov.au/sites/default/files/documents/11_2012/early_intervention_practice_guidlines.pdf*

Schertz, H. H. & Odom, S. L. (2007). Promoting joint attention in toddlers with autism: A parent-mediated approach. *Journal of Autism and Developmental Disorders*, *37*, 1562-1575.

Tschirhart, M., Christensen, R. K. & Perry, J. L. (2005). The paradox of branding and collaboration. *Public Performance & Management Review*, *29*(1), 67-84.

Tuckman, B. W. & Jensen, M. A. C. (1977). Stages of small-group development revisited. *Group & Organization Management*, *2*(4), 419-427.

van Garderen, D., Stormont, M. & Goel, N. (2012). Collaboration between general and special educators and student outcomes: A need for more research. *Psychology in the Schools*, *49*(5), 483-497.

Wahlberg, T. J. (2012). *Autism spectrum disorders: Inclusive community for the twenty-first century*. Charlotte, NC: Information Age Publishing.

In: Asperger Syndrome
Editor: Michael F. Shaughnessy

ISBN: 978-1-63463-810-4

Chapter 4

Key Barriers to Inclusion for Girls with Asperger's Syndrome at Primary School

R. Moyse and J. Porter*
University of Bath, UK

Abstract

Girls on the autistic spectrum are under-represented in the research literature and it is argued that because they present differently to boys, schools are less likely to make the adjustments needed to enable them to participate fully in the inclusive classroom. This chapter presents the findings of ethnographic case studies of three girls on the autistic spectrum at mainstream primary schools and illustrates the difficulties they experience and the ways in which this is often un-recognized. The impact on them of the hidden curriculum and the implications this might have for their right to an inclusive education is considered. Data from observations and interviews reveal the personal adjustments the girls make in response to the hidden curriculum and the ways in which these go unnoticed, effectively masking their need for support, and contributing to their underachievement in school. Lack of inclusion, particularly in terms of acceptance, had a negative impact on the girls' learning and on how they felt about school. The research also identifies a broader concept of "hidden-ness", in the attitudes and responses of the girls' teachers, peers and parents, illustrating a misunderstanding of autism in girls that contributes to a lack of support for their needs, despite their diagnosis. The study concludes that the hidden curriculum is one of a number of barriers to inclusion, resulting from the complex interaction between the girls' impairment and the environments in which they find themselves.

Keywords: Asperger's Syndrome, autism, girls, inclusion, hidden curriculum

* Email: j.porter@bath.ac.uk

Introduction

Girls on the autistic spectrum have received relatively little attention until recently (Bazelon, 2007), and the incidence of the condition is believed to be much greater in boys (Brugha et al. 2011; McPartland and Volkmar, 2013). Autism has a typically suggested male: female ratio of 4:1 (Wagner, 2006; Andersson et al. 2013), with the gender ratio previously thought to be closest where IQ is below 70 (Fombonne, 2005; Wing, 1981, cited by Gould and Ashton-Smith, 2011) and widest for those with High-Functioning Autism (HFA) or Asperger's Syndrome (AS) (Dworzynski et al. 2012). However, recent literature suggests girls who are intellectually able or appear to have better communication skills may have been under diagnosed (Kim et al. 2011; Lai et al. 2011; American Psychiatric Association, 2013). There is some evidence that the phenotype for girls is different, with this group having distinct presentations and needs (Kopp et al. 2010; Gould and Ashton-Smith, 2011; Kopp and Gillberg, 2011; Russell et al. 2011), ones that are less conspicuous than the male phenotype (Attwood et al. 2006; Gould, 2011; Solomon et al. 2012), where violent behaviour is often the trigger for teacher concern (Kopp and Gillberg, 1992; Attwood, 1999; Kopp et al. 2010).

In addition, recent research has found the ratio decreases with age (Idring et al. 2012), symptomatic of difficulties becoming greater or more apparent for girls in teenage years, suggesting an overall ratio closer to 2:1 (Kim et al. 2011; Idring et al. 2012; Kirkovski et al. 2013). There is evidence that girls acquire language earlier than boys, which may initially hide communication impairments in girls with autism (Krahn and Fenton, 2012). This is consistent with a 'reversal of trend' noted by McLennan et al. (1993, p224). They found younger girls with autism had better social skills than equivalent boys but that this pattern reversed as the girls got older. Thus whilst social difficulties for boys are more noticeable at an early age, core impairments may be hidden in younger girls (Kopp and Gillberg, 1992) but become more obvious in their teens; a time when peer-to-peer communication and interaction between girls becomes more complex. Their impairments in social interaction may therefore become more disabling for them than boys on the playground because talking is an integral characteristic of girls' play (Nichols et al. 2009; Gould and Ashton-Smith, 2011).

This may partly explain why girls are diagnosed later than boys; a recent report found that 'just 1/5 of girls had been diagnosed with AS or HFA by the age of 11, as compared to half of the males' (NAS, 2012b, p11). Girls with AS are unlikely to have a diagnosis unless they exhibit challenging behaviours (Dworzynski et al. 2012) and often only receive a diagnosis of autism in their teens or early twenties after first being referred for a secondary mental health problem (Wilkinson, 2008; Nichols et al. 2009).

Research has established that children and adults with AS are at greater risk of unhappiness and poor mental health problems than neuro-typical peers (Myles and Simpson, 2001; Portway and Johnson, 2005; Ashburner et al. 2010); girls with autism have greater emotional difficulties than boys (Mandy et al. 2012) and are more likely to have multiple anxiety disorders than their female neuro-typical peers (Kopp et al. 2010). Social Phobia, for example, has been found to have an association with teenagers with AS/HFA, and is almost twice as likely to affect girls with AS/HFA as boys (Kuusikko et al. 2008). Other disorders commonly co-morbid with autism are ADHD, OCD, sleep disorders and eating disorders, all of which may be the more obvious impairment in girls (Zucker et al. 2007; Kopp et al. 2010; Worley and Matson, 2011). Girls with autism, particularly those who are intellectually able, appear to develop coping mechanisms that mask their problems, such as becoming observers or social chameleons, or by internalising aggression and anxiety (Attwood, 2009; Solomon et al. 2012). Releasing suppressed emotions outside of school can mean extreme behavioural differences in the presentation of girls at home and at school, with parents often assessing the impact of the diagnosis more severely than teachers (Myles et al. 2007; Kopp et al. 2010; Attwood and Garnett, 2014).

There is good reason to believe that because of this different presentation these girls are less likely than boys to have their needs met in school, particularly given evidence that autistic conditions that appear less severe may impact on the level of acceptance and support received (Attwood et al. 2006; Kopp et al. 2010; Krahn and Fenton, 2012). As such, many girls with AS may be missing out on the positive early interventions that many agree are needed for the best outcomes (Wing et al. 2011; Krahn and Fenton, 2012), as well as the full benefits of an inclusive education. This chapter presents the findings of ethnographic case studies of three girls with a diagnosis of autism at mainstream primary school, and highlights the difficulties they experience plus the ways and possible reasons that these difficulties go unrecognized and unsupported. A brief discussion of inclusion in schools in England will be offered first.

Inclusion

> "For inclusion to be 'effective' all pupils must actively belong to, be welcomed by and participate in a school and community – that is, they should be fully included." (Farrell, 2004, p7)

Most children with an Autism Spectrum Condition (ASC), including AS/HFA, have been placed in mainstream schools in England since the movement towards inclusion in education began with the Education Act 1981. This was initially successful only in terms of physical integration, with the child expected to fit into the existing school culture rather than the school adjusting to meet the needs of the child (Prosser and Loxley, 2007; Feiler et al. 2012). However, legislation to ensure access and improve provision developed the principle of inclusion in the 1990's, with the Salamanca Statement by UNESCO (1994, cited by Jordan, 2008; Farrell, 2004) followed in the UK by the Code of Practice for Special Educational Needs (SEN) (1994) which considered for the first time how the needs of some SEN pupils could be met in a mainstream setting. Humphrey's 'four-pronged definition of inclusion' is used here as the most robust and relevant to this current discussion, consisting of "presence, participation, acceptance and achievement" (2008, p42).

The rights of autistic children to an inclusive education in the UK are upheld by the Equality Act 2010. This Act has meant that schools must actively make changes to support the genuine inclusion of pupils with a disability, where "disability" is defined as "a physical or mental impairment" that has a significant and 'long-term adverse effect' on daily living (Government Equalities Office, 2011, p7). Most recently, the new SEN Code of Practice (2014) has restated the UK Government's commitment to inclusive education for the disabled, "and the progressive removal of barriers to learning and participation in mainstream education" (Department for Education, 2014, p14).

There is a strong argument which suggests that disability can be reinforced by the absence of help or understanding and 'an unwillingness to adjust' on the part of others (Jordan, 2008), or this barrier can be removed:

> "Where reasonable adjustments are made the child ceases to experience disability." (Porter et al. 2012, p93)

As such disability can be seen as 'a culturally situated construct where the effect of the impairment is mediated by the adjustments and supports available in both the home and school setting' (Porter et al. 2012, p95).

A critical issue is the *impact* of the impairment or health condition, which can be disabling or have no influence at all if suitable adjustments are made (Feiler et al. 2012). Potential problems with this approach lie in who determines the impact on the child, and where the impact is measured. A child with autism may experience the impact of her condition significantly more in some environments than in others (Feiler et al. 2012, p23). Her response to this impact may only be apparent in the home environment, and be completely "invisible" to school (Porter et al. 2012, p94). The severity of the impact on girls with AS/HFA may be difficult to assess as their coping strategies are often quiet, non-combative and sometimes self-excluding (Nichols et al. 2009; Osler, 2010). This study is therefore important in drawing attention to the experience of the child, the ways in which their condition may impact on their experience of school, and on the adjustments a school might make to reduce or remove the disability.

Taking the four elements of Humphrey's definition of inclusion as central, the focus of the study was to consider the experience of girls in schools; more explicitly to examine how their difficulties impacted at different points in the school day. The particular focus lies with the hidden curriculum, "that we are not taught directly yet are assumed to know" (Myles and Simpson, 2001, p279) and to consider the impact of this on the girls and the implications this might have for inclusion.

Key Challenges at School

Arguably the most significant challenge or barrier is that presented by the requirement for almost continuous social interaction throughout each day, particularly given their seemingly milder presentation (Wagner, 2009). This may impact on every aspect of their behaviour and learning (Brown and Taylor, 1985; Jordan and Powell, 1996; Myles, 2005). In class children are expected to cooperate and collaborate, complicated interactions that require significant cognitive input (Gal et al. 2009) but which may be assumed to be within the competence of girls with AS who are verbal and intellectually able. Transitions, play times and lunch times can be even more stressful as they are "the most social and least structured" (Perepa, 2011).

Difficulties with social communication and interaction, combined with the nature of girls' play, mean that forming friendships can be particularly difficult for girls with AS. Girls typically play closely together both physically and cooperatively (Gould and Ashton-Smith, 2011). However, unspoken rules that direct play make it more difficult for girls with AS to understand how to participate in an appropriate way: they may miss out on what Grugeon calls "the essential features of the playground culture" that help shape female identity (1993, p30); they are “denied access to the very contexts in which such skills are practiced” (Jordan and Powell, 1996, p20-21). Girls with AS, wherever they sit on Wing’s behavioural continuum from “withdrawn” to “active but odd” (Jordan and Powell, 1996, p4) do want to have friends but do not have the innate skills to make it work (Attwood, 2007; Rogers, 2007; Beteta, 2009; Myles, 2013). Their joining skills are likely to be inept (Wing, 2007) and they typically lack reciprocity in play, often trying to take control as a coping strategy (Kranowitz, 2005). As a result they may experience rejection and isolation (Myles and Simpson, 1998; Wittemeyer et al. 2011) and are vulnerable to bullying (Simone, 2010; NAS 2012a).

Despite having average to high intelligence, children with AS/HFA are more likely to underachieve academically than their peers (Howlin, 2005; Ashburner et al. 2008). Problems with executive functioning, slower processing speeds plus rigid, inflexible thinking (Myles and Simpson, 2002; Attwood, 2007; Garnett et al. 2013) mean they need support to succeed in the classroom, yet this may not be obvious for girls with AS/HFA who use the strategy of internalising difficulties. Girls with AS are typically reluctant to admit when they don’t understand something (Gould and Ashton-Smith, 2011; Attwood and Garnett, 2014) and are frequently perfectionists, finding it hard to begin and complete tasks on time and to the standard they require, being excessively self-critical and afraid of failure (Ashburner et al. 2010; Gould and Ashton-Smith, 2011). This may lead to the avoidance of academic risk-taking, which may be dismissed as gender-typical.

Many children with autism also experience difficulties with processing sensory information, being hyper- or hypo-responsive, which can affect behaviour and attainment in the classroom (Kranowitz, 2005; Wing et al. 2011). Sensory Processing Disorder (SPD) has been found to impact on the ability to concentrate on cognitive tasks, for example, and hypo-responsiveness and sensory seeking behaviours have been linked to academic underachievement (Ashburner et al. 2010). Sensory sensitivities and sensory overload have also been correlated with a range of behaviours that communicate stress but challenge others, such as meltdowns, non-participation in transitions and an increase in repetitive behaviours (Myles and Simpson, 1998; Myles et al. 2013). In addition, personal hygiene and grooming activities such as daily washing, hair-brushing, teeth-cleaning and choice of clothes are sensory challenges that may be neglected as a result; which may be particularly isolating for girls due to stereotypical gender expectations around appearance (Nichols et al. 2009; Riley-Hall, 2012).

These communication and interaction difficulties, sensory sensitivities and organizational issues, combined with the challenges of interpreting the hidden curriculum of schools, mean they struggle to understand the world around them, causing greater stress and anxiety (Lawson, 1988). This in turn also impacts on their ability to learn: information retrieval is more difficult and the functioning of “the thinking part of the brain” is impaired (Myles and Southwick, 1999, p6).

Methods

The research consisted of case studies of three girls in different mainstream primary schools, utilising ethnographic methods to capture the “complexity and situatedness of behaviour” (Cohen et al. 2007, p85). This enabled the presentation and interpretation of the "uniqueness" (Cohen et al. 2007, p85) of each girl's experience, with their perspective "given voice" (Alldred, 1998, p150), using different methods to capture the "complexities of lived experience" and facilitate triangulation (Clarke and Moss, 2011, p5). Ethnography has been shown to reveal behaviours that may otherwise go undetected, "especially in the case of conformist pupils, and of girls" (Woods, 1986, p13); particularly relevant for a study such as this that looked for more subtle behaviours (Gould, 2011). Purposive sampling was used to select participants where only the age and diagnosis of the child was disclosed. The aim was for these three case studies to provide rich, detailed data consistent with a qualitative approach and supportive of the children as individuals with different experiences (Davies, 2007).

The principal method of prime data collection was non-structured non-participant observation, using a narrative system to record field notes, in order to remain objective and enable recording without preconceptions (Opie, 2004a). These procedures were informed by Clarke and Moss's (2001; 2011) "Mosaic Approach" and combined the observations with interviews, drawings, photographs and sorting activities. The aim was to "build up a picture of an individual child's experience" (Beresford et al. 2004, p181) and recognise that the girls themselves were, "Arguably…the best source of information about the ways in which schools support their learning and what barriers they encounter" (Porter, 2009, p349). Observations were initially guided by the main research question, with each girl observed continuously over a period of three consecutive days, both in the classroom and in the playground, amounting to approximately 18 hours in total. The girls were seen in core subjects each day, plus a range of other subjects and in other settings.

Semi-structured interviews were conducted with each girl's mother, class teacher and the school Special Educational Needs Co-ordinator (SENCO) to: increase validity, as per Humphrey and Lewis (2008); to discuss observations, and to give them an opportunity to comment with their own interpretations; to present their own understanding of the child, the impact of her diagnosis and how she experienced school.

Discussions with the girls were activity-led given the potential difficulties faced by any child in verbally giving full and accurate explanations to an adult, and cognisant of the additional communication issues faced by children with AS. Activities were practical and child-centred, with some selected specifically because they were already used by the girls as methods of expression and communication at home (Clarke and Moss, 2011). They used visual techniques to empower and enable the girls (Prosser and Loxley, 2007; O'Reilly, 2009), and to invite personal commentary and reactions (McLeod, 2008). A learning walk was conducted with the two younger girls, who were asked to take photographs of the places they liked to be in school. Providing them with a camera gave access to individual perceptions and provided a simple means of capturing and conveying what each girl thought was most important (Berg, 2004). Venn diagrams, drawings and mind-maps were used with all three girls to enable the sorting and prioritising of key observations displayed as symbols/PECS or text, to bring authenticity to children's views (Hayes, 2004; Prosser and Loxley, 2007; McLeod, 2008; O'Reilly, 2009). Two short sessions were spent with each girl and a partner of her choice, with a third session added in one case, to enable reflection and consolidation of meanings (Clarke and Moss, 2011).

An organisational framework was built using the text from observations in the field as it was gathered (Opie, 2004b). Initial categories of the hidden curriculum and evidence of support to access it were created. Additional categories were allowed to emerge from the data as it was collected, rather than the data collection being driven by pre-constructed classifications and preconceived assumptions (Davies, 2007, p15). Categories were revised and refined as data was re-visited or new data added (Humphrey and Lewis, 2008). Sub-categories were created for different example behaviours, referenced by line and colour-coded by girl. The process of managing and making sense of the data was aided by drawing diagrams to suggest relationships that were then checked against the data. Subsequent revisions were made if sub-categories could be combined under more salient headings, or if a sub-category or example behaviour was found to be too minor (Humphrey and Lewis, 2008).

Ethical approval for the research was granted by the University Ethics Committee prior to the collection of any data. Written consent was provided by the Head or SENCO at each school, and separately by the mother of each girl, prior to the gathering of any data. This followed written information on the purpose of the research and an opportunity to have any questions answered. A visual technique of traffic light cards was used to guide the assent of the girls to participate throughout the pair work.

Findings

Four key areas in which the hidden curriculum appeared to create difficulties for the girls were identified: class rules; working collaboratively; completing tasks and other interactions with peers. In addition, a number of modifications and coping strategies were observed being used by the girls, many of which were unnoticed or not acted upon. The hidden attitudes and actions of peers, parents and the school staff emerged as a third significant area of interest. These inform the later discussion on the impact of the hidden curriculum and of their diagnosis at school, and include observations on supports provided to manage anxiety behaviours. Contextual views of the girls accompany the research findings.

Gem

Gem was a Year 2 pupil (6-7 years) in an above average size primary school. She was referred to a paediatrician at parental request and had received a diagnosis of AS and Sensory Processing Disorder (SPD) the previous year. Her results showed that she was exceeding Age Related Expectations (ARE) in maths and reading but was below average in terms of progress and achievement in writing. She was on the school's SEN Register and she had an Individual Education Plan (IEP). She had previously attended a 10-week social skills course, and the SENCO said this support was no longer needed; she was "interacting fine". There was one 10-minute weekly intervention in place with a TA to develop her poor fine motor skills.

Interviews with Gem, her mother, teacher and the SENCO showed two areas of consensus: that she had lots of strengths (such as reading and being articulate) and that her key difficulty was her handwriting. Of her writing her teacher said, "I can't read it" while Gem said, "although my handwriting is getting better, it's still not very clear".

There were considerable differences in perspective in terms of the impact of Gem's AS at school. The breadth, frequency and severity were all scored much higher by Gem's mother than by her teacher, who believed the impact was minimal and that she had no barriers to learning: "There is nothing, I see nothing". The SENCO said that the school had not picked up any signs of impairment prior to diagnosis. Gem's mother felt that because her daughter's impairments were not always obvious it was sometimes hard to get Gem the support she needed: "because they don't see it at school, they don't acknowledge it as much of a problem".

Views varied on how much Gem enjoyed school. Her mother was positive, although she said the period of the national assessments had been very difficult with some "wobbly weeks and late arrivals". Her teacher thought Gem enjoyed school "very much"; she was very "flappy and excitable". Gem gave examples of things she enjoyed at school: lessons such as ICT (Information and Communications Technology) and science; break times and the use of equipment such as the climbing frame outside and the apparatus in the hall, and said school was "just a tiny bit over okay".

The Hidden Curriculum

Gem frequently appeared to over-react both physically and/or verbally during observations, for example making squeals of excitement with her hands over her mouth during a maths game, which marked her out from her peers.

She struggled at times to stay on task. During one maths lesson she spent 26 minutes working in a small group with a supporting adult. In this time she received 6 personal redirects but still only spent a maximum of 10 minutes on task; these 10 minutes included the time taken to get and return equipment. She struggled when teacher instructions were inconsistent, confusing or without rationale. During interview she said that the teacher using the visualiser and being able to work things out on her own helped her understand the most.

This preference for working independently was evidenced when she found it difficult to work collaboratively to reach a common agreement on, for example, a story line. Gem also made comments that illustrated her lack of social skills, such as asking a peer if her picture was better than his.

To the observer, the criteria for completing a task successfully were not always clear for Gem. Her teacher asked a lot of "test" questions: when had they drawn a silhouette before? Why was she not able to throw the javelin well? Gem was told her answers were not the ones the teacher was thinking of (although they could have been considered valid).

Gem's difficulties with the hidden curriculum were also apparent during unstructured times, when she appeared not to know how to join in with other children. During one break she jumped around a group of girls whilst on a space hopper, but she didn't join the group. On the five other unstructured periods that were observed, she played alone or alongside her peers, once picking leaves and berries for a "nest". However, unlike Scarlett or Amy, she said she enjoyed breaks. She appeared to be happy with her own company and showed no desire to communicate or collaborate with others during these times.

Personal Modifications

Gem's modifications were all apparently hidden, or noticed but not acted upon. Physical space can make social situations more challenging (Loomis, 2008) and Gem displayed a need to control it. She often discretely gave way to others as a means of managing space: she waited for her peers to finish getting things out of their trays before she approached hers; shewalked around the edge of the classroom to get to her place, turning around and finding another way through if her passage was blocked rather than pushing past or asking someone to move.

In addition Gem spent a large amount of unstructured time on her own, suggesting a need to withdraw and have her own space. During lunchtime on two days she spent 40 minutes and 37 minutes respectively on her own or not communicating and on the third day, she spent 34 of the 40 minutes on her own walking repetitively around the raised ledge surrounding the climbing frame, silently getting off and on to avoid peers who were in her path.

Gem moved almost continuously. She fiddled with blue-tac or a pencil, tapped or jiggled her feet, knelt on her seat, crouched, rocked and stood to get out of her seat. She appeared to have difficulty sitting still for any period of time and this was illustrated during a visit to a library, where the class had to sit on the carpet for 50 minutes. Gem was recorded making 31 separate movements of nine different types throughout this time.

The Influence of Others

Gem received lots of support from her maths teachers who between them provided help to her 20 times over the three maths lessons observed. This help ranged from praise and encouragement, redirecting to the task and helping with organisation to eliciting responses and checking understanding. Her class teacher made ten supportive comments or actions over three days. Gem also appeared to benefit from provisions put in place by the school to benefit all pupils, such as peer-to-peer massage and the availability of physical equipment for use by children during breaks as well as lunch times.

Gem was not always fully supported by adults who were aware of the diagnosis, however. Her teacher said that Gem was "fantastic at verbalising" in literacy but that her handwriting was almost illegible due to impairments with her fine motor skills. In terms of ARE she was underachieving and not making good progress in writing because of her difficulty in getting her thoughts onto paper, an activity in which she was engaged on a daily basis, yet no adjustments were made to support her writing during observations.

Gem had one short weekly intervention to practise "skills like cutting, colouring and strengthening my hands" (IEP); however the IEP did not state how she would be supported to improve in the classroom, other than to use a pencil grip. In addition, it appeared that no adjustment had been made to enable Gem to express her vocabulary, ideas (and organisation thereof), punctuation and grammar. The SENCO said her handwriting wasn't poor enough for her to have a scribe, and both the class teacher and the SENCO felt that using a computer for anything other than her spellings would undermine her progress in handwriting.

Her teacher told the researcher that Gem's parents had supplied a sloping cushion to use in the classroom to support her sensory needs, but that she had kept it in her cupboard because, "She's been fine all year without it". The teacher also said there was a report from the Occupational Therapist in Gem's file but that recommendations had not been carried out in the classroom. She questioned the parents' approach to discipline and how Gem could exhibit explosive behaviour at home but not school: "as far as we knew, you couldn't control it" and "I don't have to cope with anything". These remarks all imply distrust of the diagnosis or misunderstanding of the condition, and suggest that the teacher based her impact statements about Gem's diagnosis on how she was affected rather than on how Gem was affected.

Amy

Amy was a Year 3 pupil (7-8 years) at a large inner-urban primary school. She was diagnosed with AS and SPD in 2010, following a referral by the school for suspected dyspraxia. Amy was making less than satisfactory progress in writing and was underachieving in terms of ARE in maths, writing and reading.

Interviews with Amy, her mother and the school revealed two areas of consensus, which were that breaks and interacting with her peers were key difficulties. In addition, her mother, class teacher and the SENCO all stated that Amy liked to be in control, suggesting that she frequently felt out of control (Kranowitz, 2005).

The data revealed differences in the assessment of impact and required support. Amy's mother believed the frequency and severity of the impact of her AS at school was greater than the assessment made by the main class teacher, Mrs T., whilst the SENCO said that Amy required no additional support at the moment. Her mother commented that Amy's coping mechanism at home was to withdraw: "If she's feeling she's getting stressed she goes to her room". However, the SENCO stated that she had "had to discourage" the time-out space as Amy had wanted to spend a lot of time there. Amy said that it would help her if there was somewhere at school she could go to be on her own.

There were mixed views on how much Amy enjoyed school. Mrs T said that she always responded positively in lessons. Amy's mother praised the work done by Mrs T but said that her daughter didn't like coming to school: "there are too many people". Amy also mentioned the support of Mrs T; being able to stay in and do jobs was something that helped her "learn", suggesting that withdrawing enabled her to cope better with subsequent lessons. However, she said that she didn't really have any friends and was clear in her own answer: "I don't normally have that much fun usually and I don't really like coming to school".

The Hidden Curriculum

Amy's emotional responses were often too intense, such as her over-enthusiasm on finding the classroom pencils had been sharpened, and her behaviour was often inappropriate for the classroom. There were many examples of her calling out or answering questions not directed at her. During one maths lesson she called out 13 times in less than 23 minutes.

Class "rules" were not always consistent, a situation exacerbated by having two class teachers each with their own style. The way to answer a question and how to ask for help, for example, were changeable and at times confusing. Amy's inability to "muddle through" such circumstances was illustrated during a lesson to write a story (an area identified by her teachers as a weakness). Amy put her hand up to ask for help and was told to put it down because "she couldn't have a question". Seventeen minutes later she closed her book and took it over to the class teacher, who told her to sit down and, "If you have a problem put your hand up". During interview she said being given instructions 1:1 by the teacher, plus being able to see instructions as well as hear them, helped her learn the most. The structure of lessons was problematic for her, particularly science which required unsupported collaboration (her response was to dominate) and flexible thinking.

The criteria for completing a task successfully were not made explicit for Amy. She was pleased to be first to finish in almost every lesson, stating "When you finish first it means like you've done more work than anybody". Her teacher asked children to do their "best work", but this was not further defined. In a science lesson Amy's group got a different but equally valid result to their teacher, but the teacher did not accept or discuss an alternative answer.

Her impairments in social interaction were most apparent and least supported in the playground. Amy's play was physical, aggressive and non gender-typical. Her behaviour was very controlling: she forced herself between others, pushed a peer so hard he nearly fell into some mud, and then pretended to tie him to the perimeter fence with a skipping rope. Her interactions usually had an unhappy outcome: she upset her peers or became distressed herself during four of the six breaks and lunch times she was observed.

Personal Modifications

Amy's biggest modification appeared to be her attempts to conceal from others when she didn't understand. Her work outcomes were rarely checked at the time; field notes evidenced two lessons when her written work was checked during the session, but seven when it wasn't. She tried to hide her work from her peers, handed it in without having it checked, wrote illegibly in tiny letters on her whiteboard or rubbed her writing out before the teacher had seen it. She kept looking busy rather than asking for help by picking up reading books or extension activities: in one literacy lesson she spent 15 minutes on the writing task and 22 minutes on four different maths extension activities, only two of which she attempted correctly.

Amy exhibited behaviours consistent with high levels of background anxiety (Attwood and Garnett, 2014). She sought opportunities to organise equipment and to be the one to hand out any items required for a lesson. She frequently tried to organise the people around her, during both structured and unstructured times. This behaviour included reprimanding classmates for breaking the rule of standing on a chair and instructing peers how to move around during a pre-school Parkour session. She chewed her fingers most of the time, and fiddled with pencils and bits of thread, leant or rubbed against furniture and sat with her chair legs pressing into her feet. During a learning walk with the researcher she said that whilst fiddling helped her to concentrate and made her "happier", "It doesn't make the teacher very happy! It makes the teacher shout at me".

Amy also made modifications in response to the challenges of the school day in ways that were enabled or legitimised by their teachers, often to manage unstructured periods. She was not where she was supposed to be for 9 of the 12 observed transitions to/from the playground. She came in early from all three lunch times, although she was the first to go out. She delayed going out for break by (incorrectly) giving out books for the next lesson and always came into the classroom early.

Amy managed her own space by positioning herself at the front of a line or on the same place on the carpet, and extended this to her wider environment, for example by getting up to close the classroom door if it was left open. She chose how long to spend on a task: in ICT she spent 5 minutes on the task and 23 minutes experimenting and instructing her neighbours. She had regular jobs such as collecting and returning hi-visibility jackets for the walk to the swimming pool, and getting the fruit snack ready for the class at break. However, these jobs impacted on her learning time: in one maths lesson she spent as much time cutting the stalks off tomatoes for break as she did on the maths activity.

The Influence of Others

In terms of positive support measures, Mrs T. often checked that Amy understood a task and provided her with individual instructions and prompts. Mrs T. (and on one occasion her phonics teacher) also worked on her self-esteem, praising her for excellent work, trying hard and being helpful. Environmental measures such as the outside climbing equipment provided for all pupils and a range of visual supports in the classroom were well used by Amy.

There were some negative attitudes at school, however. There was a disparity between the information her mother received about the support given to Amy, and the reality. She was unaware that some support strategies (such as the time-out space) had been removed. Some teachers felt the mother used the diagnosis "as an excuse" and one said: "I don't think she can cope [with Amy]".

Interviews with Amy's class teachers and the SENCO illustrated that they were aware of the difficulties she faced at school and the teachers recognised that these challenges were often unsupported: "We have children who have more needs". However, they were unclear about her diagnosis, and thought her sensory-seeking behaviour was ADHD.

Not all adults that came into contact with the Amy were aware of her diagnosis. Until recently, lunchtime controllers had not been told that Amy had AS and "just thought she was naughty". Her class teacher, Mrs T., said there was a tension between keeping certain things confidential and sharing information, but felt that in situations such as these the knowledge should be cascaded through the school to better support the child.

Her peers rarely interacted with her during lessons and whose responses to her were sometimes nonverbal. During interview she talked about not liking lunchtimes or playing, about being bullied, and listed crying as one of the things that she does during these times. When she was very tearful and upset during lunch time one day, she approached a number of children for comfort and support, but each one drifted away from her rather than engaged. One of the reasons Amy gave for not liking school was that she didn't have any friends.

Scarlett

Scarlett was a Y6 pupil (10-11 years) atttending a slightly above average size primary school, and had been there for four years. She was diagnosed with autism seven years previously, following a referral by her Health Visitor and the nursery she attended at the time, when the family was living in a large city in the north of England. Since then she has had a Statement of Need for 1:1 support (currently 15 hours/week). She was intellectually high-functioning, had made expected progress and was on target to meet or exceed National assessment targets that year. Scarlett had not been told of her diagnosis.

Interviews with her mother, class teacher (Mrs D), TA and the SENCO revealed a comprehensive shared understanding of Scarlett's strengths and difficulties. All said that social situations and unstructured times (including unstructured lessons) were the most challenging for her, as did Scarlett, and they recognised the impact they had on her learning: "If she's had a difficult break or lunch she can find it hard to concentrate" (Mrs D). Her mother, Mrs D and TA noted she had high levels of anxiety, with school staff stating this impacted on her concentration, confidence and performance in some subjects, notably maths. They all said that her coping strategy was to internalise her anxiety and retreat: "If she's not feeling comfortable she does withdraw," and she "tends to work more by herself" (Mrs D).

The only area of disagreement was whether or not Scarlett should be told of her diagnosis. Her mother felt that telling her would make her "more stressed, more anxious"; the SENCO felt "she ought to be aware". Mrs D was sure she was already aware: "I don't believe she doesn't know. She's a very bright girl". In terms of her enjoyment of school, both her mother and Mrs D thought she was generally happy. Her mother was highly supportive of Mrs D and the school. Scarlett's feelings about school appeared to be directly linked to the quality of her social interactions and were not so positive: "I treat everyone as normal people but they don't, they seem to like ignore me. I feel like I don't exist here".

The Hidden Curriculum

Scarlett frequently over-reacted both physically and/or verbally in the classroom during observations; her exuberance at being able to plant a few oats on a school trip suggesting she was not aware of the intensity of emotional responses appropriate in the classroom. She also displayed behaviours that were inappropriate in the classroom, such as responding personally to all instructions directed at the class. During interview she said she got annoyed if expected to muddle through, though having the ability to work out what was going on was least visibly a problem for Scarlett. She struggled to work collaboratively, preferring to work on her own ideas when asked to be part of the Y6 production advertising team rather than interact with her peers, or to direct a member of the group. She said she learnt best when she could work on her own, or when the teacher modeled something for her. Interviews with her teacher and with her confirmed that she struggled with particular lesson structures, specifically when she was required to work as part of a team and notably in science:

> "I like science but sometimes I find it a bit boring because I don't really get included in much stuff…sometimes no one listens to me, so um, we don't really work, they don't really like my ideas, so I like working on my own most of the time."

Interacting with her peers was one of Scarlett's biggest hurdles and it was in the playground that her impairments in social interaction were most apparent and least supported. During breaks she sat quietly on the edge of a group, apparently listening but not joining in. She said that she often felt "lonely" and "left on her own" by her peers; "they don't want me they want somebody else".

Personal Modifications

Scarlett made some modifications that may have been hidden from others, for example often discretely giving way to others as a means of managing her space. She waited for other people to finish collecting items from the cloakroom before getting hers, and on her school trip she always walked around the back of a group instead of jostling with her classmates to find a position where she could see clearly.

Some of her feelings were completely hidden from the researcher, despite careful observation, and were only revealed during interview, reinforcing the importance of pupil voice. It was clear, for example, that anxiety was a big issue for Scarlett, and that she tried to hide it. It was also apparent to others that her self-esteem was low: "Lots of people say I say negative stuff about myself because I always think negative about myself. I don't think positive too much". What she effectively internalized, however, was her frustration and displeasure at being ignored, enduring wet play, having to muddle through or working in a team, as evidenced by a classification activity of support strategies for learning.

Scarlett exhibited some modifications that were not noticed, or noticed but not acted upon, such as controlling behaviours towards people and things. On one occasion Scarlett systematically checked and restocked the pen pots in her classroom for 18 minutes just before she left for a visit to JF, the secondary school she was to attend in September, so that each table had the same of everything. Her mother later said that Scarlett was apprehensive about the visit. Scarlett also made many small, frequent movements. She was given a piece of wool during an activity on her school trip, which she then fiddled with through the day. In school she fiddled with her hair or small things such as the hem of a piece of clothing or a pencil, and swung, jiggled or tapped her legs. Fidget tools were provided in the classroom, but she didn't use them. During interview she said, "They help me, yes, but no one really lets me have a turn that much, so, so I don't really bother with it anymore, I just fiddle with what I have". Her mother later told the researcher that Scarlett played with her hair when she was nervous.

Some modifications were enabled or legitimised by her teachers. She was allowed to stay in and do jobs or go to the library at break time, and to go into the corridor on her own to vote. The relief from lessons felt by most children at break time was not true for Scarlett; it was the inverse: "I feel sad when I get left out and then I feel happy when I'm doing lessons because it just gets my mind off break time and lunch time". A major conflict for Scarlett was that she wanted to be included and yet one of her main coping strategies when she was unhappy or got stressed was to withdraw, thus excluding herself.

The Influence of Others

The classroom culture of which Scarlett was part was particularly autism-friendly. The style of teaching was inclusive and aware, with academic measures such as providing a rationale as well as explicit instructions, modelling expectations and monitoring understanding, plus the approach was consistent (Myles et al. 2004). Some environmental adjustments had been made and opportunities were taken to build Scarlett's self-esteem, such as praising her poster for a play in front of the class.

However, the secrecy of her diagnosis meant that some causes of anxiety could not be fully addressed. This was particularly notable with her visit to JF, which was (unknown to her) an additional visit for all Y6 pupils with autism in the secondary school's catchment. She travelled in a taxi with two (male) classmates with a known diagnosis of autism, though her mother said Scarlett did not want to and did not understand why she had been grouped with two peers with autism. In terms of the influence of her peers, Scarlett said she found social interactions at break "confusing" and "upsetting".

Discussion

Despite apparent differences in the profile of the girls, the case studies revealed how all three girls experienced problems navigating the hidden curriculum in and out of the classroom (Brown and Taylor, 1985), suggesting it was a significant barrier to inclusion. In direct contrast to common recommendations for teachers of autistic children (Myles and

Simpson, 1998; Lanning, 2000; NAS, 2011), class rules were sometimes inconsistent, expectations were not always made explicit and comprehension was often unchecked. National advice is that teachers should provide structure both in and out of the classroom so that school is a less chaotic place (Humphrey, 2008; Perepa, 2011; NAS, 2012b). In class this should include "consistency, routines, clear specification of task and performance requirements, clearly understood behavioral expectations" (Simpson et al. 2011, p13). All three girls did best when the teachers were "consistent in the way they structure their classrooms and predictable in the way they act" (Myles and Simpson, 1998, p67).

Participation in "the activities of the school" (IPSEA, 2011, p12) incorporates inclusion during breaks, lunch times and transitions, and the findings showed that these unstructured periods were problematic for all three girls. Social interaction with peers was challenging for all of them, and two felt bullied and isolated. This identified the importance of decoding "the unwritten rules of girls' social interactions" (Gould and Ashton-Smith, 2011, p38), including "the behaviours that constitute bullying" and what to do about them (Simpson et al. 2011, p11). Children on the spectrum cannot "muddle through" but need "to be told and shown" (Brown and Taylor, 1985, p9). These children do not learn by "osmosis" (Jordan and Powell, 1996, p15) but need to be taught cognitively (Elliot et al. 1985; Jordan and Powell, 1996; Myles, 2005), and thus the skills to interact and form friendships with other children must also be taught.

Previous research has recommended that social skills be taught in real-life, meaningful settings (Koegel at al, 1982; Arendt et al. 1985) with "girl-orientated personal, social skills classes" (Gould and Ashton-Smith, 2011, p38) - to which none of the girls in this study had access. There is a logical argument for these skills to be taught to autistic girls with their peers during these times, as this is both when girls with AS are at their most vulnerable, and when neuro-typical girls develop their own skills (Jordan and Powell, 1996). Hidden rules governing interaction and friendship can thus be identified with the input of positive female peer role models and can be practiced in the correct context. Research by Ferraioli and Harris (2011) suggests that their participation in such programmes may also result in neuro-typical peers having better attitudes towards pupils with autism, and a greater assessment of their competence. Teaching social skills and building independence during unstructured periods would require significant changes to staffing (and mindsets), but could be done through more flexible deployment of teaching assistants trained in individual-specific strategies to achieve this.

Research suggests teaching about the nature of female friendships can also be done effectively through a partnership between home and school. In one case presented by Chamberlain et al. (2007), the mother of a girl with AS worked with the mother of a popular female peer to identify ways in which she could be encouraged to reach out to the autistic girl, the school speech therapist wrote social scripts for her about how to join play, the teacher identified the way girls greeted each other in the morning and that was practiced at home and in speech therapy, and the mother practiced these social interactions with her daughter at home.

All three girls displayed a need to withdraw and rebalance during unstructured periods, "a real need for solitude" (Sainsbury in NAS, 2012b, p2), and this must be enabled and balanced with the need to develop social skills. Time alone to recharge is particularly pertinent for girls, of whom there are more expectations to interact socially (Faherty, 2006) and who therefore may be more prone to social fatigue. This need to withdraw was met in part by two schools, though the opportunity to withdraw was based on the individual teacher's willingness to allow this: Mrs D, Amy's teacher, chose to let her come into the classroom before the end of the lunch break, but noted that this time was officially a non-contact period for her and that her next teacher would be "...under no obligation to give up her own time". These observations point to the importance of a whole school policy governing such support.

A key unexpected finding of this research was that a diagnosis was not sufficient in itself to ensure support for full access to the curriculum for these girls, despite evidence of their social isolation and rejection, anxiety behaviours, and academic under-achievement in some subjects. Impairments caused by AS/HFA that were found in this study to be disabling could sometimes be explained by a lack of teacher knowledge or awareness (Symes and Humphrey, 2011; Keane et al. 2012). Not all teachers fully understood the diagnosis and its implications for teaching and learning, and this was a considerable barrier to inclusion for two of the girls. Where there were inconsistencies in school rules and teacher expectations, or other evidence of the hidden curriculum, staff did not always appear to be aware of this, or of the implications. They were thus not always in a position to notice when something presented a challenge to their pupil.

Teachers did not all recognise subtle behavioural signs of anxiety in girls such as nail-biting and chewing, "withdrawal/escape" and "repetitive behaviours" (Ozsivadjian et al. 2012, p113), or know how best to support the girls. This needs to change if the under-achievement and mental health issues described by Kuusikko et al. (2008), Nichols et al. (2009) and Ashburner et al. (2010) are to be avoided in adolescence. Support for mental health is known to improve the "quality of life" of children with autism (Ghaziuddin, 2005, p9) and can be fostered in school by building self-esteem, confidence and emotional well-being (Myles and Simpson, 2001), promoting peer understanding and tolerance (Myles and Simpson, 1998; Wagner, 2006; Humphrey, 2008), and providing opportunities for the girls to do that at which they excel: good practice for all pupils.

Given the complexity of the autistic spectrum, it is not surprising that teachers lack full understanding. Generally they do not have sufficient training to tackle the range of conditions they may meet in the classroom (Attwood, 2007; Mooney et al. 2010; Autism Education Trust, 2011; Szatmari, 2011), and this lack of skills and knowledge constitutes an additional barrier. This study found that each girl had different preferences for what helped them learn, indicating a need for teachers to understand how autism affects each individual. Appropriate targeted training is therefore key (Leblanc et al. 2009; McCullough, 2014) and has been cited by parents in some studies as the most important element in order to enable their pupils in mainstream (Barnard et al. 2000; Jindal-Snape et al. 2005).

Research has confirmed the importance of including modules on how to teach children with autism in University teacher training programmes (Leblanc, et al. 2009). Once in the school environment, however, targeted training for all staff working with a particular child has been found to be much more effective than generic autism awareness for all staff in the school (Ferraioli and Harris, 2011; Symes and Humphrey, 2011; Humphrey and Symes, 2013), and enables an understanding of how to meet the child's needs which is based on her individual symptoms and particular strengths (Jindal-Snape et al. 2005). The effectiveness of a teacher has been found to increase according to the amount of autism-specific experience they have, suggesting that training should include "high quality and co-ordinated field experiences" (Simpson et al. 2011, p6) at schools with proven expertise and wide experience in teaching autistic children.

Of concern was the lack of attention given by teachers in two schools to the knowledge of parents. Elsewhere it has been argued that parent views are central to understanding the impact of an impairment or health condition (Porter et al. 2013), and yet the involvement of parents has been found to be "heavily influenced by the extent to which school professionals actively encourage…their contributions" (Simpson et al. 2011, p7). Here it was evident that where the severity of impact of the impairment was not assessed by the class teacher or the SENCO at as high a level as the mother, a negative or dismissive attitude was detected towards both the parenting style and the diagnosis. This suggests that the teachers concerned based their impact statements about a girl's diagnosis on how it affected others in the classroom including them, rather than on the impact on the child.

In consequence some teachers also failed to access other relevant information, including post-diagnosis recommendations from external professionals, which would have supported inclusion. Suggestions of how to meet a child's sensory needs in school, for example, can be provided by Occupational Therapists to "reduce anxiety and clumsiness and improve…social participation" (Kranowitz, 2005, p33); this information was available but not used by one school.

The findings support earlier studies that demonstrate the importance of hearing the pupil's voice and of the school and parents sharing experiences so that there is a common understanding (Porter et al. 2013). Impact on the pupil cannot be judged by the impact the pupil has on the teacher, particularly when the teacher is also responsible for providing any support.

The implications of assessment of impact for the provision of reasonable adjustments and school-based support are significant, though new legislation in England in the form of the Special Educational Needs Code of Practice (2014) may address this issue. Education, health and social care services must work together where this "improves the quality of special educational provision" (Department for Education, 2014, p13), and schools must "ensure decisions are informed by the insights of parents and those of children and young people themselves" (Department for Education, 2014, p14), thus recognising the expertise and knowledge parents have of their own child.

The lack of drive from teachers to understand these girls and how they learn was a concern in two schools, and the attitude of teachers and how they viewed their role identified as another barrier to inclusion. The findings illustrate the potential impact of a teacher's interactions on a child with AS/HFA, of the classroom and playground environments they set up, and of their belief over whether they had "ultimate responsibility for ensuring students with ASDs' learning and participation" (Humphrey and Lewis, 2008, p135).

Acceptance by peers was another issue for all three girls. The research found that Gem went out at break and lunch times but played in isolation, but that she appeared to be accepted by her peers. Amy was frequently rejected by her peers and Scarlett said she did not feel accepted by her peers, experiences that were upsetting for both of these girls. Interestingly, the relationship between a teacher and an autistic child has been found to impact on the level of social acceptance from a child's peers (Humphrey and Symes, 2011), suggesting this needs to be good in order for pupils to also be accepting.

Successful inclusion therefore requires a positive approach from teachers (Humphrey and Symes, 2011). Work by Leblanc et al. (2009) found that training has a positive impact on attitudes, whilst later research has shown that "experience, knowledge, [and] attitudes were all interrelated" (Segall and Campbell, 2012, p1164), lending further weight to the importance of professional development as detailed above. Critically though, inclusion can not result from the work of a few members of staff, or by inserting a module into the curriculum, but must rather be adopted by the whole school as an ethos that forms an integral part of everything they do:

> "Without a shift in the whole organizations's attitude and approach it will fail children with autism and Aspergers Syndrome" (Barnard et al. 2000, p12).

Finally, and significantly, the research found that the presentation and behaviour of the girls may contribute to a lack of understanding in schools and subsequent lack of support. It has already been argued that girls are often relatively inconspicuous compared to boys in school (Attwood et al. 2006; Solomon et al. 2012; Attwood and Garnett, 2014), although Amy demonstrated there is a broader phenotype. Despite outward differences, though, all three girls shared core similarities, notably in terms of "masking" impairment as a coping strategy (Solomon et al. 2012), in line with the previously identified coping strategies of internalising and hiding.

These findings demonstrate the girls made personal adjustments that were very discrete or that they tried to hide, and that these effectively influenced the perception that others had of the impact of autism on their lives at school. An assessment of needs for a girl with autism therefore needs to be clearly differentiated from the impact that girl has on the teacher or on the rest of the class. Without this, a vicious circle is created with the girls making more and more of their own modifications to compensate for the lack of support provided in school, which in turn leads teachers to think that the impact of autism is small and thus less support needs to be provided (Figure I).

The findings, when considered against Humphrey and Lewis's (2008) four-pronged definition of presence, participation, acceptance and achievement, suggest that the experience of none of the three girls would fully meet the criteria for inclusion.

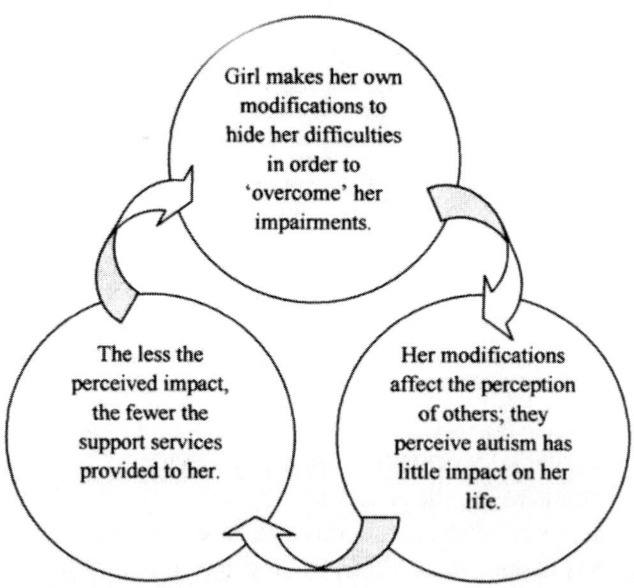

Figure 1. Modifications by the girls.

The research found that Gem was withdrawn for one intervention each week, which she appeared to enjoy, and was otherwise present in the classroom and appeared to be accepted by her peers. She was exceeding Age Related Expectations ARE in mathematics and reading, but did not appear to do so in writing or in "social and emotional domains" (Humphrey and Lewis, 2008, p133). She did go out at break and lunch times but played in isolation; participation was also an issue during group work in class, though (as the youngest girl in the sample) it is difficult to assess whether the behaviour was developmentally age-related.

Amy had the least inclusive experience, partly because she often chose to remove herself and effectively self-exclude. She was frequently not where she was supposed to be, did not engage with set tasks with the objective of learning and understanding, and chose when to participate and when to complete an activity. Some of these behaviours were enabled by teachers to her detriment, for example by not checking her understanding and allowing her to do inappropriate extension activities; others such as legitimizing her coming into the classroom early from lunch were beneficial but only in the short-term. She was underachieving academically, socially and emotionally, and was not accepted by many of her peers.

Scarlett was achieving at or above ARE but did not choose the most challenging tasks to complete), suggesting she may have been under-achieving. She was always present in the classroom. However, she sometimes self-excluded at break times or by choosing to work alone, she was segregated with two boys with autism for a visit to their secondary school, which confused her, and she did not feel accepted or understood by her peers; a situation that was clearly distressing for her.

It is noteworthy that the girl having the least inclusive experience of school was underperforming the most, and was demonstrably the least happy. All children have a right to an inclusive education and this means access to all aspects of the curriculum, including those that may be termed the "hidden curriculum."

Conclusion

The case studies of three very different individuals help to extend what is already known about the presentation of girls with AS/HFA. Some research has been done on girls at secondary school; this study highlights the need for further research at primary school level. Whilst it is not possible to generalise the results across all girls with AS/HFA at primary school, they offer insights into the experiences of girls, and also illuminate for teachers some of the unseen challenges faced by girls with AS/HFA as well as how they may be supported (Carrington and Graham, 2001; Humphrey and Lewis, 2008).

From a legal standpoint, UK schools are required to make "reasonable adjustments" (EHRC, 2012, p4) to meet the needs of all their disabled pupils, and earlier legislation requires schools "to use their best endeavours to:…ensure that the child engages in the activities of the school together with children who do not have special educational needs" (IPSEA, 2011, p1-2). Without an understanding of AS/HFA and how the condition impacts on the way these girls learn, schools that do not address the hidden curriculum may also by default be failing to provide an inclusive education.

This research found that the hidden curriculum creates a significant barrier to inclusion for girls with AS/HFA, as earlier defined by Humphrey's (2008) four elements. They do not learn intuitively so must be taught implicit rules and school culture. However, their coping mechanisms of masking and internalizing difficulties and anxieties make them vulnerable to not having their needs met in school, even with a formal diagnosis. The research found that the hidden attitudes of teachers and peers contributed further to a lack of inclusion, as did their limited knowledge. This is significant because unless teachers understand the need to address the hidden curriculum due to the way girls with autism learn, they are also at risk of not teaching the known curriculum in a way these girls can access. Targeted training, more flexible deployment of staff and a whole school ethos of acceptance are required to overcome these barriers.

The key barriers to inclusion for these girls therefore mirror how we might understand disability: as a complex interaction between the girls' difficulties, the environments in which they find themselves, their strategies for coping and the teachers responses – or not – to these factors. The girls and their parents provide important insights that facilitate teachers in understanding the complexity of this interaction. However this also needs to be set within a whole-school culture of acceptance, of neuro-diversity as "normal", if true inclusion is to be achieved as it is the interaction between the impairment and the environment that defines whether autism is disabling for these girls at school.

References

Alldred, P. (1998). Ethnography and discourse analysis: dilemmas in representing the voices of children. *In*: J. Ribbens, and R. Edwards (Eds.), Feminist Dilemmas in Qualitative Research: Public Knowledge and Private Lives (pp147-170). London: Sage.

American Psychiatric Association. (2013). Diagnostic and statistical manual of mental disorders 5. American Psychiatric Association.

Andersson, G. W., Gillberg, C. and Miniscalco, C. (2013). Pre-school children with suspected autism spectrum disorders: Do girls and boys have the same profiles? *Research in Developmental Disabilities,* 34(1), 413-422.

Arendt, L., Connelly, L. and Connelly, M. (1985). Language and Communication. *In*: Association of Heads and Teachers of Adults and Children with Autism (Eds), *The Special Curricular Needs of Autistic Children* (pp20-25). Loughborough: AHTACA.

Ashburner, J., Ziviani, J. and Rodger, S. (2008). Sensory Processing and Classroom Emotional, Behavioral, and Educational Outcomes in Children with Autism Spectrum Disorder. *American Journal of Occupational Therapy*, 62(5), 564-573.

Ashburner, J., Ziviani, J. and Rodger, S. (2010). Surviving in the mainstream: Capacity of children with autism spectrum disorders to perform academically and regulate their emotions and behavior at school. *Research in Autism Spectrum Disorders,* 4(1), 18-27.

Attwood, T. (1999). The Pattern of Abilities and Development of Girls with Asperger's Syndrome. Retrieved February 26, 2012 from http://www.aspergerfoundation.org.uk/infosheets/ta_girls.pdf.

Attwood, T. (2007). The Complete Guide to Asperger's Syndrome. London: Jessica Kingsley Publishers.

Attwood, T. (2009). Ask Tony: Girls with Asperger's. Retrieved February 7, 2012, from http://www.autismhangout.com/news-reports/feature-programs.asp?id2=123.

Attwood, T., Faherty, C., Wagner, S., Wrobel, M., Bolick, T., Myers, J.M., Snyder, R. and Grandin, T. (2006). Aspergers and Girls. Arlington, Texas: Future Horizons.

Attwood, T., and Garnett, M. (2014, April). Assessing the Traits of Asperger's Syndrome. Presentation at the 'Attwood on Asperger's and Autism' Conference, Autism Oxford.

Autism Education Trust. (2011). Educational Provision and Outcomes for People on the Autism Spectrum. Retrieved November 15, 2011, from http://www.autismeducationtrust.org.uk/Resources/Outcomes.aspx.

Barnard, J., Prior, A., and Potter, D. (2000). Inclusion and autism: is it working? London: National Autistic Society.

Bazelon, E. (2007). What Autistic Girls Are Made Of. Retrieved April 25, 2012, from http://www.poacnova.org/news_uploads/2578/New%20York%20Times%20Magazine%208-5-07%20--%20What%20Autistic%20Girls%20AreMade%20Of.pdf.

Beresford, B., Tozer, R., Rabiee, P. and Sloper, P. (2004). Developing an approach to involving children with autistic spectrum disorders in a social care research project. *British Journal of Learning Disabilities,* 32(4), 180-185.

Berg, B. L. (2004). Qualitative Research Methods for the Social Sciences. Boston: Pearson Education.

Beteta, L. M. (2009). A phenomenological study of the lived experiences of adolescent females with Asperger Syndrome. Retrieved January 22, 2012, from http://gradworks.umi.com/33/42/3342492.html.

Brown, W. and Taylor, G. (1985). Impaired Relationships and Self Image. *In*: Association of Heads and Teachers of Adults and Children with Autism (Eds), *The Special Curricular Needs of Autistic Children* (pp6-13). Loughborough: AHTACA.

Brugha, T. S., McManus, S., Bankart, J., Scott, F., Purdon, S., Smith, J. et al. (2011). Epidemiology of autism spectrum disorders in adults in the community in England. *Arch Gen Psychiatry,* 68(5) 459-65.

Carrington, S. and Graham, L. (2001). Perceptions of school by two teenage boys and their mothers: a qualitative study. *Autism,* 5(1) 37-48.

Chamberlain, Kasari and Rotheram-Fuller (2007). Involvement or Isolation? The Social Networks of Children with Autism in Regular Classrooms. *Journal of Autism and Developmental Disorders*, 37 (2) pp230-242.

Clarke, A. and Moss, P. (2001). Listening to Children: The Mosaic Approach. London: National Children's Bureau.

Clarke, A. and Moss, P. (2011). Listening to Young Children: The Mosaic Approach (2nd edn). London: National Children's Bureau.

Cohen, L., Manion, L. and Morrison, K. (2007). Research Methods in Education. London: Routledge.

Davies, M.B. (2007). Doing a Successful Research Project. Basingstoke: Palgrave Macmillan.

Department for Education (2014) Special educational needs and disability code of practice: 0 to 25 years. Statutory guidance for organisations which work with and support children and young people with special educational needs or disabilities. Retrieved July 6, 2014, from https://www.gov.uk/government/uploads/system/uploads/attachment_data/file /325875/SEND-Code_of_Practice-June2014.pdf.

Dworzynski, K., Ronald, A., Bolton, P., and Happé, F. (2012). How Different Are Girls and Boys Above and Below the Diagnostic Threshold for Autism Spectrum Disorders? Journal of the American Academy of Child & Adolescent Psychiatry, 51(8), 788-797.

EHRC. (2012). Reasonable Adjustments for Disabled Pupils. Retrieved January 31, 2013, from http://www.equalityhumanrights.com/uploaded_files/EqualityAct/reasonable_adjustments_for_disabled_pupils_guidance_pdf.pdf.

Elliot, A., Farrell, M., Jordan, R., and Parker, S. (1985). Cognitive Skills. *In:* Association of Heads and Teachers of Adults and Children with Autism (Eds), *The Special Curricular Needs of Autistic Children* (pp26-31). Loughborough: AHTACA.

Faherty, C. (2006). Asperger's Syndrome in Women: A different set of challenges? *In*: T. Attwood, C. Faherty, S. Wagner, M. Wrobel, T. Bolick, J. M. Myers, R. Snyder, and T. Grandin (Eds), Aspergers and Girls (pp9-14). Arlington, Texas: Future Horizons.

Farrell, P. T. (2004). School psychologists, making inclusion a reality for all. *School Psychology International,* 25(1) 5-19.

Feiler, A., Porter, J., Daniels, H., Georgeson, J., Hacker, J. and Martin, S. (2012). The use and usefulness of a parent questionnaire to help schools identify disability. *Journal of Research in Special Educational Needs,* 12(1), 22-27.

Ferraioli and Harris (2011). Effective Inclusion of Students on the Autism Spectrum. *Journal of Contemporary Psychotherapy*, 41 (1) pp19-28.

Fombonne, E. (2005). Epidemiological studies of pervasive developmental disorder. *In*: F. Volkmar, R. Paul, A. Klin, D. Cohen (Eds), Handbook of Autism and Pervasive Developmental Disorders (pp42-69). Hoboken, NJ: Wiley.

Gal, E., Bauminger, N., Goren-Bar, D., Pianesi, F., Stock, O., Zancanaro, M. and Weiss, P.L. (2009). Enhancing Social Communication of Children with High- Functioning Autism with a Co-located Interface. *AI & Society*, 24(1) 75-84.

Garnett, M., Attwood, T., Peterson, C. and Kelly, A. B. (2013). Autism spectrum conditions among children and adolescents: a new profiling tool. *Australian Journal of Psychology,* 65 (4) 206-213.

Ghaziuddin, M. (2005). Mental Health Aspects of Autism and Asperger Syndrome. Jessica Kingsley Publishers: London.

Gould, J. (2011). Missed Diagnosis or Misdiagnosis? Retrieved April 21, 2012, from http://vimeo.com/27015431

Gould, J. and Ashton-Smith, J. (2011). Missed diagnosis or misdiagnosis? Girls and women on the autistic spectrum. GAP, 12(1), 34-41.

Government Equalities Office. (2011). Equality Act 2010: Guidance. Retrieved January 31, 2013, from http://www.homeoffice.gov.uk/publications/equalities/equality-act-publications/equality-act-guidance/disability-definition?view=Binary.

Grugeon, E. (1993). Gender implications of children's play- ground culture. In: P. Woods and M. Hammersley (Eds), Gender and Ethnicity in Schools: Ethnographic Accounts (pp11-33). London: Routledge & Open University Press.

Hayes, J. (2004). Visual Reviews: How to include pupils with learning difficulties in their educational reviews. *Support for Learning,* 19(4), 175-180.

Howlin, P. (2005). Outcomes in Autism Spectrum Disorders. *In*: P. Volkmar and C. Klin (Eds), Handbook of Autism and Pervasive Developmental Disorders (3rd edition, pp201-222). Hoboken, NJ: Wiley.

Humphrey, N. (2008). Including pupils with autistic spectrum disorders in mainstream schools. *Support for Learning*, 23(1), 41–47.

Humphrey, N. and Lewis, S. (2008). What does 'inclusion' mean for pupils on the autistic spectrum in mainstream secondary schools? *Journal of Research in Special Educational Needs*, 8(3), 132-140.

Humphrey and Symes (2013). Inclusive education for pupils with autistic spectrum disorders in secondary mainstream schools: teacher attitudes, experience and knowledge. *International Journal of Inclusive Education*, 17 (1) pp32-46.

Idring, S., Rai, D., Dal, H., Dalman, C., Sturm, H., Zander, E., Lee, B.K., Serlachius, E. and Magnusson, C. (2012) Autism Spectrum Disorders in the Stockholm Youth Cohort: Design, Prevalence and Validity. *PLoS ONE* 7(7): e41280. doi:10.1371/journal.pone.0041280.

IPSEA. (2011). Governor Training: Duties towards children with SEN. Retrieved November 27, 2012, from http://www.ipsea.org.uk/AssetLibrary/Downloadable%20documents/Govenors%20SEN%20duties%20-%20ipsea%20training%20Jan%202011%20(2).pdf

Jindal-Snape, D., Douglas, W., Topping, K.J., Kerr, C. and Smith, E.F. (2005). Effective provision for children with autistic spectrum disorder: Perceptions of parents and professionals. *International Journal of Special Education*, 20 (1) pp77-87.

Jordan, R. (2008). Autism Spectrum Disorders: a challenge and a model for inclusion in education. *British Journal of Special Education*, 35(1), 11-15.

Jordan, R. and Powell, S. (1996). Understanding and Teaching Children with Autism. Chichester: John Wiley.

Keane, E.,Aldridge, F.J., Costley, D. & Clark, T. (2012). Students with autism in regular classes: a long-term follow-up study of a satellite class transition model. *International Journal of Inclusive Education*, (16) 1001-1017.

Kim, Y.S., Leventhal, B.L., Koh, Y.J., Fombonne, E., Laska, E., Lim, E.C., Cheon, K.A., Kim, S.J., Kim, Y.K., Lee, H., Song, D.H. and Grinker, R. R. (2011). Prevalence of Autism Spectrum Disorders in a Total Population Sample. *American Journal of Psychiatry*, 168 (9) 904-12.

Kirkovski, M., Enticott, P. G., and Fitzgerald, P. B. (2013). A Review of the Role of Female Gender in Autism Spectrum Disorders. *Journal of Autism and Developmental Disorders*, 43 (11) 2584-2603.

Koegel, R.L., Rincover, A and Egel, A.L. (1982). *Educating and Understanding Autistic Children*. San Diego: College-Hill Press.

Kopp, S. and Gillberg, C. (1992). Girls with Social Deficits and Learning Problems: Autism, Atypical Asperger Syndrome or a Variant of These Conditions. *European Child and Adolescent Psychiatry,* 1(2), 89-99.

Kopp, S. and Gillberg, C. (2011). The Autism Spectrum Screening Questionnaire (ASSQ)-Revised Extended Version (ASSQ-REV): An instrument for better capturing the autism phenotype in girls? A preliminary study involving 191 clinical cases and community controls. *Research in Developmental Disabilities*, 32(6) 2875-2888.

Kopp, S., Kelly, K. B. and Gillberg, C. (2010). Girls with Social and/or Attention Deficits: A Descriptive Study of 100 Clinic Attenders. *Journal of Attention Disorders,* 14(2), 167-181.

Krahn, T. M. and Fenton, A. (2012). The Extreme Male Brain Theory of Autism and the Potential Adverse Effects for Boys and Girls with Autism. *Bioethical Enquiry,* 9, 93-103.

Kranowitz, C.S. (2005). The Out-of-Sync Child. New York: Penguin.

Kuusikko, S., Pollock-Wurman, E., Jussila, K., Carter, A.S., Mattila, M-J., Ebeling, H., Pauls, D.L. and Moilanen, I. (2008). Social Anxiety in High-functioning Children and Adolescents with Autism and Asperger Syndrome. *Journal of Autism and Developmental Disorders,* 38(9) 1697-1709.

Lai, M-C., Lombardo, M.V., Pasco. G., Ruigrok, A.N.V., Wheelwright, S.J., Sadek, S.A., Chakrabarti, B., MRC AIMS Consortium, Baron-Cohen, S. (2011). A Behavioral Comparison of Male and Female Adults with High Functioning Autism Spectrum Conditions. *PLoS ONE* 6(6): e20835. doi:10.1371/journal.pone.0020835.

Lanning, L. (2000). People with Autism: The Effectiveness of the TEACCH Programme. Norwich: UEA.

Lawson, W. (1988). Understanding and Working with the Spectrum of Autism. London: Jessica Kingsley Publishers.

Leblanc, L., Richardson. W. and Burns, K.A. (2009). Autism Spectrum Disorders and the Inclusive Classroom: Effective Training to Enhance Knowledge of ASD and Evidence-based Practices. *Teacher Education and Special Education, 32*(2) pp166-179.

Loomis, J.W. (2008). Staying in the Game: Providing Social Opportunities for Children and Adolescents with Autism Spectrum Disorders and other Developmental Disabilities. Shawnee Mission, KS: AAPC Publishing.

Mandy, W., Chilvers, R., Chowdhury, U., Salter, G., Seigal, A. and Skuse, D. (2012). Sex Differences in Autism Spectrum Disorder: Evidence from a Large Sample of Children and Adolescents. *Journal of Autism and Developmental Disorders*, 42 (7) 1304-1313.

McCullough, M.I. (2014). Teacher Self-Efficacy in Working with Children with Autism in the General Education Classroom. Retrieved June 28, 2014, from http://gradworks.umi.com/36/14/3614480.html.

McLeod, A. (2008). Listening to Children: A Practitioner's Guide. London: Jessica Kingsley Publishers.

McPartland, J.C. and Volkmar, F.R. (2013). Asperger Syndrome and its Relationships to Autism. *In*: J.D. Buxbaum and P.R. Hof (Eds), *The Neuroscience of Autism Spectrum Disorders* (pp55-68). Oxford: Elsevier Press.

Mooney, A., Statham, J., Brady, L-M., Lewis, J., Gill, C., Henshall, A., Willmott, N., Owen, C., Evans, K. (2010). Special Educational Needs and Disability: Understanding Local Variation in Prevalence, Service Provision and Support. Retrieved April 1, 2013, from https://www.education.gov.uk/publications/eOrderingDownload/DCSF-RB211ES.pdf

Myles, B. S. (2005). The Cycle of Tantrums, Rage, and Meltdowns in Children and Youth with Asperger Syndrome, High-Functioning Autism, and Related Disabilities. Retrieved March 3, 2013, from http://www.isec2005.org.uk/isec/abstracts/papers_m/myles_b.shtml

Myles, B. S., 2013. Building Social Skills Instruction in Children with Asperger Syndrome. In: R. W. DuCharne and T. P. Gullotta (Eds), Asperger Syndrome: A Guide for Professionals and Families (pp91-111). New York: Springer Books.

Myles, B. S., Hudson, J., Lee, H. J., Smith, S. M., Tien, K-C., Chou, Y-C. and Swanson, T. C. (2007). A Large-Scale Study of the Characteristics of Asperger Syndrome. *Education and Training in Developmental Disabilities*, 42(4), 448–459.

Myles, B. S. and Simpson, R. L. (1998). Asperger Syndrome: A Guide for Educators and Parents. Austin, Texas: PRO-ED.

Myles, B. S. and Simpson, R. L. (2001). Understanding the Hidden Curriculum: An Essential Social Skill for Children and Youth with Asperger Syndrome. *Intervention in School and Clinic*, 36(5) 279-286.

Myles, B. S. and Simpson, R. L. (2002). Asperger Syndrome: An overview of characteristics. *Focus on Autism and other Developmental Disabilities*, 17(3), 132-7.

Myles, B.S. and Southwick, J. (1999). Asperger Syndrome and Difficult Moments. Kansas, Texas: APC.

Myles, B. S., Trautman, M. L. and Schelvan, R. L. (2004). The Hidden Curriculum: Practical Solutions for Understanding Unstated Rules in Social Situations. Shawnee Mission: APC.

Myles, B. S., Trautman, M. L. and Schelvan, R. L. (2013). The Hidden Curriculum for Understanding Unstated Rules in Social Situations for Adolescents and Young Adults. Kansas: AAPC Publishing.

NAS. (2011). Classroom and Playground: Support for Children with Autistic Spectrum Disorders. Retrieved April 12, 2014, from http://www.autism.org.uk/working-with/education/educational-professionals-in-schools/lessons-and-breaktimes/education-classroom-and-playground-support-for-children-with-autism-spectrum-disorders.aspx

NAS. (2012a). Anti-Bullying Week Press Release. Retrieved December 3, 2012, from http://www.autism.org.uk/news-and-events/media-centre/press-releases/press-releases-nov-2012.aspx.

NAS. (2012b). Understanding Difficulties at Break Time and Lunchtime. Retrieved March 16, 2013, from http://www.autism.org.uk/working-with/education/educational-professionals-in-schools/lessons-and-breaktimes/education-understanding-difficulties-at-break-time-and-lunchtime.aspx

Nichols, S., Moravcik, G. M., & Tetenbaum, S. P. (2009). Girls Growing up on the Autism Spectrum. London: Jessica Kingsley Publishers.

Opie, C. (2004a). Research Procedures. In: C. Opie (Ed), Doing Educational Research (pp95-129). London: Sage.

Opie, C. (2004b). Presenting Data. In: C. Opie (Ed), Doing Educational Research (pp130-161). London: Sage.

O'Reilly, K. (2009). Key Concepts in Ethnography. London: Sage.

Osler, A., Street, C., Lall, M. and Vincent, K. (2002). Not a Problem? Girls and School Exclusion. Retrieved January 17, 2012, from http://marielall.com/Files/Reports /NPI%20schools%20exclusions%20girls.pdf.

Ozsivadjian, A., Knott, F. and Magiati, I. (2012). Parent and child perspectives on the nature of anxiety in children and young people with autism spectrum disorders: a focus group study. *Autism,* 16(2), 107-121.

Perepa, P. (2011). Classroom and playground: support for children with autism spectrum disorders. Retrieved June 27, 2012, from http://www.autism.org.uk/working-with/education/educational-professionals-in-schools/lessons-and-breaktimes/education-classroom-and-playground-support-for-children-with-autism-spectrum-disorders.aspx.

Porter, J. (2009). Missing out? Challenges to hearing the views of all children on the barriers and supports to learning. Education 3-13: International Journal of Primary, Elementary and Early Years Education, 37(4), 349-360.

Porter, J., Daniels, H., Martin, S., Hacker, J., Feiler, A. & Georgeson, J. (2012). Supporting schools in identifying and safeguarding the needs of disabled children: the challenges for data collection. *Educational Review*, 64(1), 77-98.

Porter, J., Georgeson, J., Daniels, H., Martin, S. and Feiler, A. (2013). Reasonable adjustments for disabled pupils: what support *do* parents want for their child? European Journal of Special Needs Education, 28(1), 1-18.

Porter J. (in press). Understanding and Responding to the Experiences of Disability. London: Routledge.

Portway, S.M., and Johnson, B. (2005). Do you know I have Asperger's Syndrome? Risks of a non-obvious disability. *Health Risk & Society*, 7(1), 73-83.

Prosser, J. and Loxley, A. (2007). Enhancing the Contribution of Visual Methods to Inclusive Education. *Journal of Research in Special Educational Needs,* 7(1), 55-68.

Riley-Hall, E. (2012). Parenting Girls on the Autism Spectrum. London: Jessica Kingsley Publishers.

Rogers, C. (2007). Experiencing an 'Inclusive' Education: Parents and Their Children with 'Special Educational Needs'. *British Journal of Sociology of Education,* 28(1), 55-68.

Russell, G., Steer. C. and Golding, J. (2011). Social and demographic factors that influence the diagnosis of autistic spectrum disorders. *Social Psychiatric Epidemiology.* 46 (12) 1283-1293.

Segall, M. J., & Campbell, J. M. (2012). Factors relating to education professionals' classroom practices for the inclusion of students with autism spectrum disorders. Research in Autism Spectrum Disorders, 6(3) pp1156-1167. Simone, R. (2010). Aspergirls. London: Jessica Kingsley Publishers.

Simpson, R.L., Mundschenk, N.A. and Heflin, L.J. (2011). Issues, policies and recommendations for improving the education of learners with autistic spectrum disorders. *Journal of Disability Policy Studies,* 22 (1), *3-17.*

Solomon, M., Miller, M., Taylor, S., Hinshaw, S. and Carter, C. (2012). Autism Symptoms and Internalizing Psychopathology in Girls and Boys with Autism Spectrum Disorders. *Journal of Autism and Developmental Disorders*, 42(1), 48-59.

Symes, W. and Humphrey, N. (2011). School factors that facilitate or hinder the ability of teaching assistants to effectively support pupils with autism spectrum conditions (ASDs) in mainstream secondary schools. *Journal of Research in Special Educational Needs*, 11(3), 153-161.

Szatmari, P. (2011). New Recommendations on Autism Spectrum Disorder. *BMJ,* 342: d2456.

Wagner, S. (2006). Educating the Female Student with Asperger's. *In:* T. Attwood, C. Faherty, S. Wagner, M. Wrobel, T. Bolick, J. M. Myers, R. Snyder, and T. Grandin (Eds), Asperger's and Girls (pp15-32). Arlington, Texas: Future Horizons.

Wilkinson, L. A. (2008). The Gender Gap in Asperger Syndrome: Where are the Girls? TEACHING Exceptional Children Plus, 4(4). Retrieved April 17, 2013, from http://journals.cec.sped.org/tecplus/vol4/iss4/art3/

Wing, L. (1981). Language, Social, and Cognitive Impairments in Autism and Severe Mental Retardation. *Journal of Autism and Developmental Disorders*, 11(1), 31-44.

Wing, L. (2007). Children with Autistic Spectrum Disorders. *In*: R. Cigman (Ed), Included or Excluded? The Challenge of the Mainstream for some SEN Children (pp.23-33). Oxon: Routledge.

Wing, L., Gould, J. and Gillberg, C. (2011). Autism spectrum disorders in the DSM-V: Better or worse than the DSM-IV? Research in Developmental Disabilities, 32 (2) 768-773.

Wittemeyer, K., Charman, T., Cusack, J., Guldberg, K., Hastings, R., Howlin, P., MacNab, N., Parsons, S., Pellicano, L and Slonims, V. (2011). Educational Provision and Outcomes for People on the Autistic Spectrum Retrieved November 15, 2011, from http://www.autismeducationtrust.org.uk/Resources/Outcomes.aspx.

Woods, P. (1986). Inside Schools: Ethnography in Educational Research. London: Routledge & Kegan Paul.

Worley, J. A., and Matson, J. L. (2011). Psychiatric Symptoms in Children Diagnosed with an Autism Spectrum Disorder: An Examination of Gender Differences. *Research in Autism Spectrum Disorders*, 5(3) 1086-1091.

Zucker, N. L., Losh, M. Bulik, C. M., LaBar, K. S., Piven, J. and Pelphrey, K. A. (2007). Anorexia Nervosa and Autism Spectrum Disorders. *Psychological Bulletin,* 133(6) 976-1006.

In: Asperger Syndrome
Editor: Michael F. Shaughnessy
ISBN: 978-1-63463-810-4

Chapter 5

QEEG/LORETA Electrical Imaging and Z-score LORETA Neurofeedback: New Approach to Diagnosis and Therapy of Autistic Spectrum Disorders (ASD)

J. Lucas Koberda, MD, PhD*
Tallahassee Neuro Balance Center, Tallahassee, FL, US

Abstract

Introduction of QEEG/LORETA brain imaging has improved our diagnostic ability in neuropsychiatric practice by identification of dysregulated cortical areas implicated in patient's symptoms. Additional use of LORETA Z-score neurofeedback (NFB) enables us to directly target these areas of dysregulation in order to improve associated with them symptoms. Based on approximately 250 patients treated in our clinic with Z-score LORETA NFB and suffering from different neuropsychiatric conditions a detailed analysis of our cases of ASD are presented. Specific areas of cortical dysregulation identified by QEEG/LORETA are described as well as results of computerized cognitive testing are presented. Follow up findings of QEEG/LORETA electrical imaging after NFB and computerized cognitive testing indicating NFB mediated cognitive enhancement are shown.

Keywords: EEG, QEEG, LORETA, electrical imaging, Asperger Syndrome, Autistic Spectrum Disorder, neurofeedback

* Corresponding author: E-mail: JLKoberda@yahoo.com; www.TallahasseeNeuroBalanceCenter.com

Introduction

Autism is a neurodevelopmental disorder characterized by impaired *social interaction* and *communication*, and by restricted and repetitive behavior. It is one of three recognized disorders in the *autism spectrum* disorders (ASD), the other two being *Asperger Syndrome* (AS), which lacks delays in cognitive development and language, and Pervasive *Developmental Disorder, not otherwise specified* (PDD-NOS), which is diagnosed when the full set of criteria for autism or Asperger Syndrome are not met (AMA, 2000).

The *prevalence* of autism is about 1–2 per 1,000 people worldwide, and the *Centers for Disease Control and Prevention* (CDC) report 11 per 1,000 children in the United States are diagnosed with ASD as of 2008. Parents usually notice signs in the first two years of their child's life. *Early behavioral* or cognitive intervention can help autistic children gain self-care, social, and communication skills. Results of quantitative EEG (QEEG) showed generally increased delta-theta activity in frontal region of the brain. Changes in QEEG pattern appeared to be in a non-linear correlation with maturational processes (Pop-Jordanova et al. 2010). More recently Coben and his group have defined ASD as a disorder of abnormal neuronal connectivity-his research has shown a combination of mixed over and under-connectivity that is at the heart of the primary symptoms of this disorder (Coben et al. 2014).

Asperger Syndrome (AS), frequently considered as mild form of ASD is characterized by significant difficulties in social interaction, alongside restricted and repetitive patterns of behavior and interests. It differs from other autism spectrum disorders by its relative preservation of *linguistic* and *cognitive development.* Although not required for diagnosis, physical clumsiness and atypical use of language are frequently reported. The syndrome was named after the Austrian pediatrician *Hans Asperger* who, in 1944, studied and described children in his practice who lacked *nonverbal communication* skills, demonstrated limited *empathy* with their *peers*, and were physically clumsy. Individuals with AS experience difficulties in basic elements of social interaction, which may include a failure to develop friendships or to seek shared enjoyments or achievements with others. Stereotyped and repetitive motor behaviors are a core part of the diagnosis of AS and other ASDs. They include hand movements such as flapping or twisting, and complex whole-body movements. Echolalia has also been observed in individuals with AS. There is no single treatment, and the effectiveness of particular interventions is supported by only limited data. Intervention is aimed at improving symptoms and function. The mainstay of management is *behavioral therapy*, focusing on specific deficits to address poor communication skills, obsessive or repetitive routines, and physical clumsiness. Most children improve as they mature to adulthood, but social and communication difficulties may persist. More recently, neurofeedback (NFB) has been reported as a potential treatment modality which could benefit ASD individuals.

ASD and Epilepsy

A number of studies suggest that seizures affect a high proportion of children with autism spectrum disorder (ASD). The reported prevalence of epilepsy in ASD ranges from 5 to 38%, which is clearly higher than the 1–2% prevalence in the general childhood population (Frye et al. 2013). A recent larger cross-sectional study suggests that the prevalence of epilepsy is 12.5% in children with ASD aged 2–17 years with this prevalence clearly highest for adolescents (Viscidi et al. 2013). In addition, the prevalence of treatment-resistant epilepsy in children with ASD is believed to be higher than in the general childhood population (Sansa et al. 2011).

Two meta-analyses suggest that NFB can reduce seizures in a majority of patients, even in patients with otherwise uncontrolled epilepsy (Sterman B, 2000, and Tan et al. 2009). Research suggests that NFB may be an effective form of cognitive therapy for children with ASD (Coben et al. 2010). Other case studies suggest that it also may be helpful for in control of seizure disorders in ASD (Coben et al. 2009).

Neuroeedback in ASD

NFB training, which involves operant conditioning of self-regulatory processes involved in the production of endogenous brain rhythms, can lead to functional changes in neural networks (Pineda, 2008). NFB training offers the opportunity to operantly condition these dynamics and examine the consequences of such training on cognition and behavior (Lubar, 1997). Other author's studies suggest that NFB training has behavioral and electrophysiological consequences for children with ASD. Mu suppression, which is typically absent in these children (Oberman et al., 2005) recovers following 10 weeks of mu rhythm NFB training compared to those receiving placebo training. At the same time, positive changes in attention, impulsivity, and other assessments of behavior assessed by parents also change. NFB has been successfully utilized for over 40 years in both the clinic and in research. However, support for the efficacy of NFB in ASD is limited and based primarily on a few case studies, rather than randomized, controlled, blinded studies (Lilienfeld, 2005). Specifically relevant to this issue are two published investigations involving NFB with autistic children. Jarusiewicz (2003) administered NFB to 12 autistic children and reported an average of 26% improvement on autistic symptoms as rated by the Autism Treatment Evaluation Checklist (ATEC), compared to 3% improvement in a matched placebo group. Sichel (1995) in a single case study using NFB, reported improvement in all diagnostic dimensions for autism. In a recent study completed at Behavioral Science Institute, Radboud University Nijmegen, NFB among patients called "EEG-regulators" produced no statistically significant reductions of symptoms of ASD but they showed significant improvement in cognitive flexibility (Kouijzer et al. 2013). Thomson's also reported very good results of large group (over 150 patients) of ASD patients subjected to NFB therapy (Thompson et al. 2010). Specifically the positive outcomes of decreased symptoms of Asperger's and ADHD (including a decrease in difficulties with attention, anxiety, aprosodias, and social functioning) plus improved academic and intellectual functioning, provided preliminary support for the use of NFB as a helpful component of effective intervention in people with ASD. The average gain for the Full Scale IQ score was 9 points in this study (Thompson et. al. 2010).

More recently the neuroscience group from University of Montreal has shown that NFB therapy is able to induce white and grey matter changes (Ghaziri et al. 2013). Therefore these neuronal modulations may be responsible for majority of cognitive benefits attributed to NFB therapy.

Methods Including Low Resolution Electromagnetic Tomography Analysis (LORETA) Imaging

Deymed Truscan 32 (Deymed Diagnostic, Payette, ID) EEG equipment was combined with Neuroguide (Applied Neuroscience, Inc.) software. The NFB protocol included surface and LORETA (NF1/NFB2) feedback, in an alternating protocol while focusing on a symptom checklist including: attention deficits, concentration problems, executive function problems and short-term memory. A commercially available computerized neurocognitive testing battery was used for the initial and follow up assessments of many patients (NeuroTrax Corp, Bellaire, TX). Neurotrax Corporation cognitive testing is a computerized neuropsychological assessment where the patient is compared to aged and education matched healthy controls where mean is 100 and the standard deviation is 15. QEEG analysis was completed using commercially available Neuroguide software (Applied Neuroscience, Inc.) and previously recorded 19 channel digital EEG.

Approximately 1-3 minutes of artifact-free eyes closed EEG segments were selected after previously recording EEG with the Deymed, Truscan 32, (Deymed Diagnostic, Payette, ID) and subjected to further QEEG analysis. NFB therapy consisted of 30-minute sessions once or twice a week using auditory and/or visual feedback.

To localize the cortical sources of scalp EEG activity we used low resolution electromagnetic tomography analysis (Pascual-Marqui RD et al. 1994). The low resolution electromagnetic tomography analysis (LORETA) method is a discrete, three-dimensional (3D) distributed, linear, inverse solution. The smoothing constraints in LORETA endows the tomography with the property of low localization errors to test point sources, albeit with low spatial resolution (i.e., neighboring neuronal sources will be highly correlated (Pascual-Marqui RD et al. 1994). The LORETA inverse solution corresponds to the 3D distribution of electrical neuronal activity that features a maximum similarity (i.e., maximum synchronization), in term of orientation and strength, between neuronal populations in adjacent voxels. The imaging is therefore particularly tuned towards synchronized brain activities as they occur, e.g., in spreading oscillatory activations. Since LORETA takes explicitly into account that scalp electric potentials are determined up to an arbitrary additive constant, the final LORETA solution is independent of the electrical reference used. Deep structures such as the anterior cingulate cortex, (Pizzagalli D et al. 2001) insula and mesial temporal lobes (Zumsteg D et al. 2006) can be correctly localized with LORETA.

Z-Score LORETA Imaging and Biofeedback

EEG biofeedback also called neurofeedback (NFB), is a type of biofeedback that uses real-time displays of EEG to illustrate brain activity and teach self-regulation.

NFB has resulted in a wide range of biofeedback approaches, but many good clinical outcomes required more than 50 to 80 sessions.

However, the goal is to achieve good clinical outcome in fewer sessions. Real-time fMRI biofeedback can achieve modification of blood flow and regulate the activity in specific brain regions, e.g., amygdala in patients with depression (Young KD et al. 2014). Despite the fact that fMRI signal-Blood Oxygen Level Dependent (BOLD) is an indirect measure, there is growing evidence for a strong correlation between the BOLD signal and electrical brain activity (Sitaram R et al. 2007). Studies have characterized the relationship between localized increases in neuronal activity and the corresponding increase in BOLD (Logothetis et al. 2001, Shmuel et al. 2006), making it possible to interpret positive functional responses in terms of neural changes. However, high costs associated with fMRI use are considered as one of prohibitive causes limiting its use in clinical settings. Therefore, LORETA EEG-biofeedback, which can be applied with relatively low cost at any clinic, seems to be superior for accomplishing a self-regulation of the brain.

In the 1990s, a new form of EEG biofeedback (Z-score biofeedback) was suggested, in which real-time comparisons to an age matched reference population of healthy or normal subjects are used as a guide or "compass" to increase specificity and provide a uniform direction and threshold for the biofeedback process (Thatcher, 2012). Prior to Z score biofeedback clinicians had to guess about what threshold to set for a given frequency or location to trigger the feedback signal or reinforcer signal (Thatcher, 2012).

Z score biofeedback greatly simplifies and standardizes EEG biofeedback by reducing many different metrics (absolute power, relative power, ratios, coherence, phase) to a single or common metric of the Z score or a standard deviation with respect to the EEG from a group of age matched healthy normal subjects (Thatcher, 2012).

Surface Z scores improve specificity by isolating dysregulated locations and rhythms, especially when using the Laplacian transform and LORETA Z scores are even more specific. For example, LORETA Z score biofeedback often also produces results in one 20 minute session because EEG source localization has accuracies of about 1 cm to 3 cm and thus is much more specific than is surface EEG (Thatcher RW, 2012).

In Z-Score NFB, a real-time comparison to an age-matched population of healthy subjects is used for data acquisition, simplifying protocol generation and allowing clinicians to target modules and hubs that indicate dysregulation and instability in networks related to symptoms (Thatcher, 2013). Z-score NFB increases specificity in operant conditioning, providing a guide that links extreme Z-score outliers to symptoms, and then reinforcing Z-score shifts toward states of greater homeostasis and stability. The goal is increased efficiency of information processing in brain networks related to the patient's symptoms (Thatcher, 2013).

A recently introduced method called Low Resolution Electromagnetic Tomography (LORETA) Z-score NFB is capable of targeting specific dysregulated anatomical structures, many of which are in deep cortical locations (Koberda et al., 2013; Thatcher, 2013). For example, the insula and anterior cingulate have been identified as potential NFB target sites for improving pain control in patients who display electrical dysregulation of these areas (Koberda et al. 2013).

In this chapter I would like to review our experience and preliminary results in therapy of patients with ASD with use of LORETA Z-score NFB.

Out of approximately 250 patients who have completed LORETA Z-score NFB therapy due to variety of neuropsychiatric disorders 10 patients were diagnosed with ASD (see Table 1. for details). All our patients reported subjective improvement of their symptoms during and after NFB therapy. Most of the patients were found to have objective improvements of QEEG abnormalities identified before NFB therapy initiation. The most frequent finding on QEEG testing was frontal increase in beta power with frequently associated increase in frontal or temporal elevation of delta or theta power. Only a few patients were able to complete computerized cognitive testing before and after NFB. After completion of NFB the cognitive testing revealed marked cognitive enhancement in most of the patients tested (Table 1). More detailed analysis of these individuals will be presented below.

Review of Cases

Case 1

This is a 12 year old autistic boy who's family was interested in trying NFB as therapeutic modality. He had practically no speech output except occasional single words, was restless and fidgety. MRI of the brain was normal. His Neurotrax cognitive testing was grossly abnormal with low memory score of 25.7 and attention score of 39.7. QEEG showed marked increase of central and temporal beta power (Figure 1A) and LORETA demonstrated anterior cingulate (BA-24) electrical dysregulation (Figure 1B).

This patient completed only five NFB sessions (due to insurance termination) after which his family noticed some improvement in his behavior, mostly noticing him being less restless. In addition, after five NFB sessions, reduction of excessive beta activity was noted.

Table 1. Shows ASD patient's demographics and other clinical information

Age and Diagnosis	Subjective improvement	Objective Improvement QEEG	Cognitive testing Neurotrax	Number of NFB sessions
1. 12 yo M	Yes	Yes	N/A	5
2. 15 yo M	Yes	Yes	N/A	10
3. 5 yo M	Yes	Yes	N/A	56
4. 6 yo M	Yes	Yes	Yes-Improved	87
5. 23 yo M	Yes	Yes	N/A	47
6. 18 yo M	Yes	Yes	N/A	51
7. 14 yo F	Yes	No	N/A	7
8. 12 yo M	Yes	Yes	NA	8
9. 18 yo M	Yes	Yes	Yes-improved	25
10. 14 yo M	Yes	Yes	Yes-improved	35

M-male, F-female.

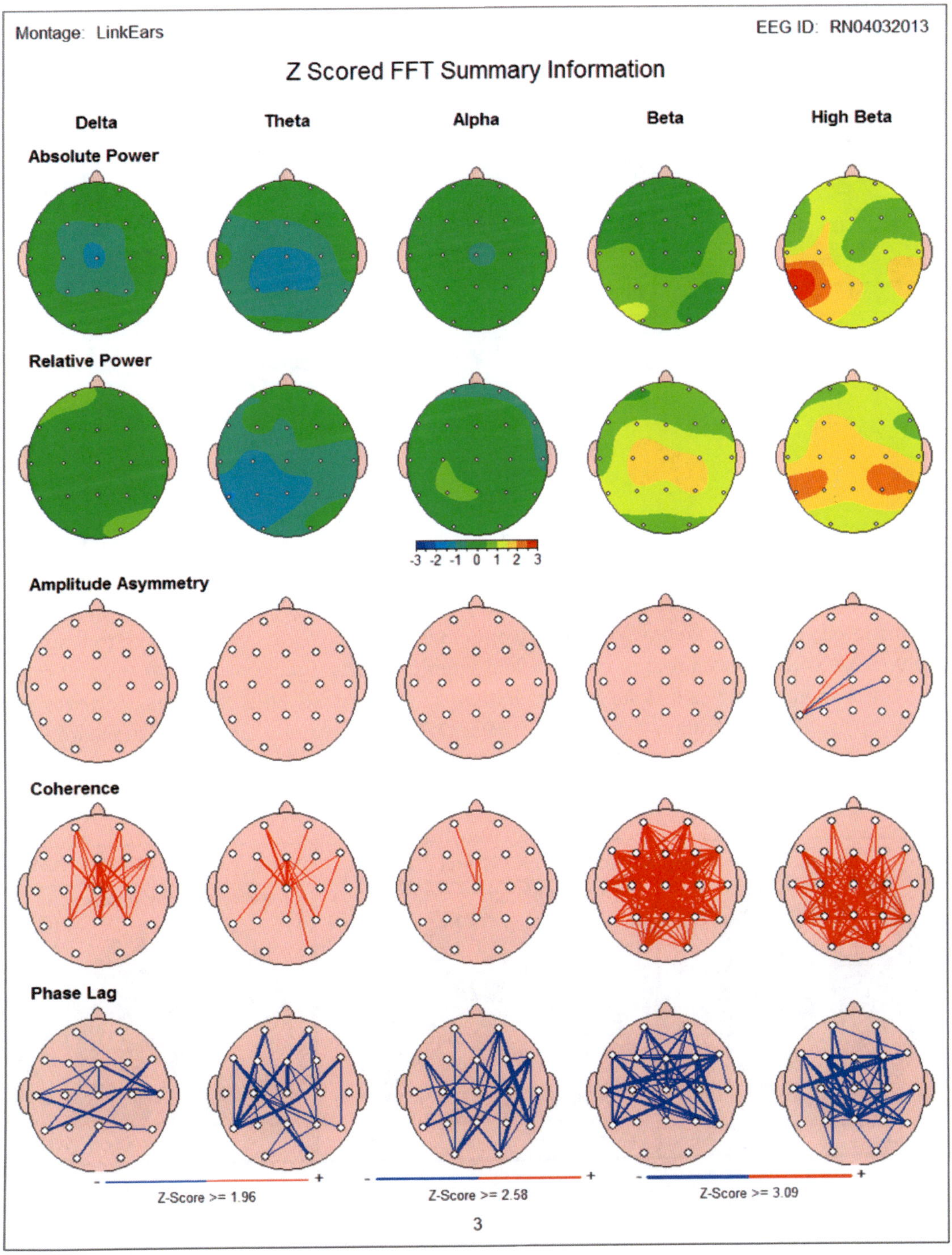

Figure 1A. This is 12 year old boy with ASD. QEEG shows increased central and temporal beta power (in red).

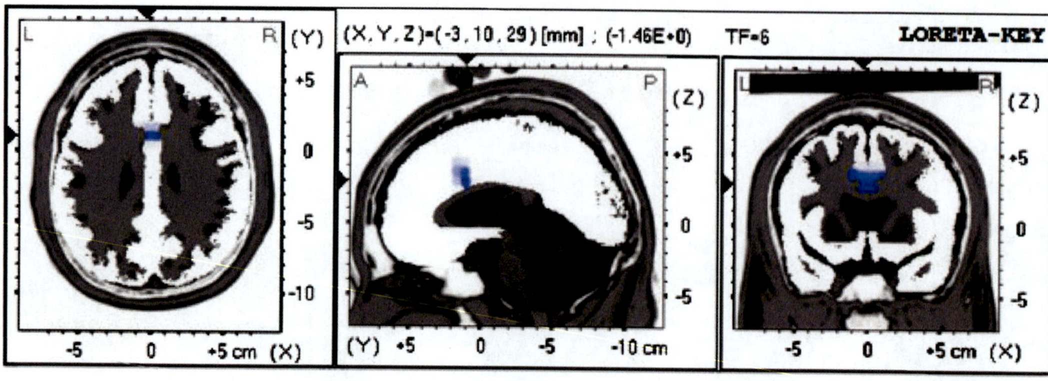

Figure 1B. 12 year old autistic boy-LORETA showed area (in blue) of anterior cingulate electrical dysregulation in theta frequency.

Case 2

This is 15 year old boy with history of Asperger Syndrome associated with ADHD and behavioral problems including anger control. His cognitive profile showed Global Cognitive Score (GCS)-90.5 with weakness in memory-87.8 and verbal function-68.7. LORETA demonstrated (Figure 2) area of electrical dysregulation in the right frontal lobe Brodmann's area 9 (BA-9) which has a role in memory and other cognitive functions. QEEG showed mild increase in frontal beta and delta power. Patient completed 10 NFB sessions, however no follow up cognitive testing was accomplished. Overall his family and the patient noticed some subjective improvement in his cognition. QEEG recorded after NFB also showed some improvement of previously identified abnormalities.

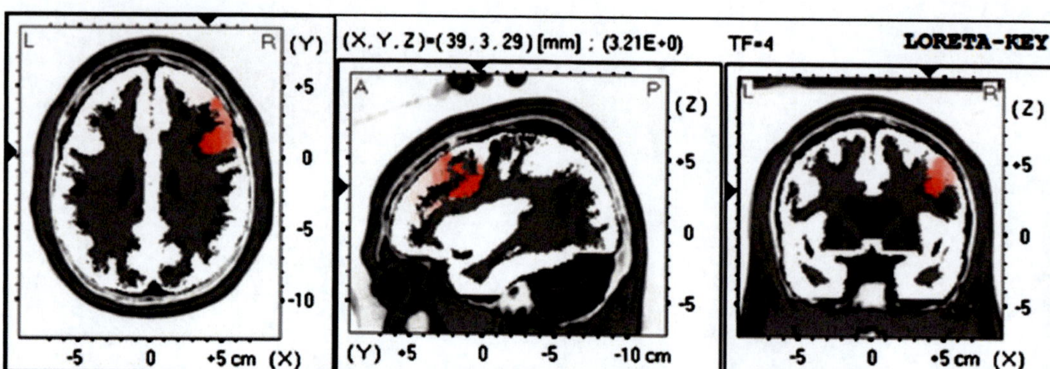

Figure 2. 15 year old male with AS. LORETA showed electrical dysregulation of BA-9 (in red) in delta frequency.

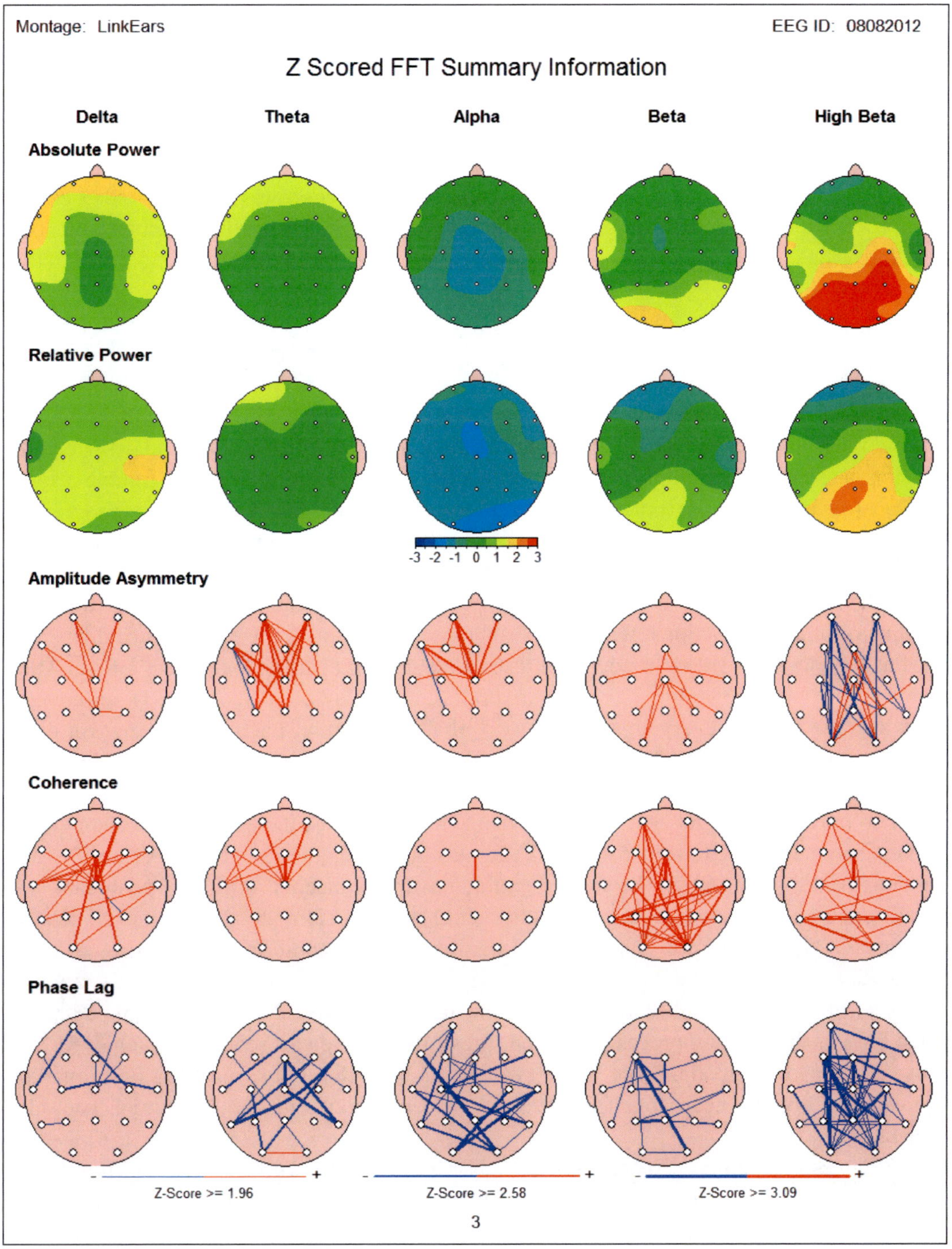

Figure 3. 5 year old boy with autism. QEEG showed elevated central and occipital beta power (in red) and frontal increase in delta power.

Case 3

This is 5 year old boy who started NFB due to family request. He was diagnosed with autism with no verbal output and was able to follow simple commands. Due to young age and cognitive limitations, he was not able to complete Neurotrax testing. QEEG showed central and occipital increase in beta power, as well as frontal elevation of delta power (Figure 3). Patient has completed 56 NFB sessions, with mild improvement of his behavior and cognitive function (increased vocalization). His repeated QEEG revealed reduction of beta overexpression.

Case 4

An eight year old male with Asperger Syndrome associated with Attention Deficit Hyperactivity Disorder (ADHD) came with his mother for an examination. She described his problems at school, including learning and behavioral difficulties. He had trouble paying attention (resulting in poor grades), and was enrolled in the special education program at school. He had a history of speech delay, clumsiness, and was often fidgety and unable to sit still. The mother reported neither prior medical problems nor pregnancy complications. During the examination, he often interrupted and squirmed around in his chair; he was alert and able to follow instructions. Before NFB therapy was initiated, the eight-year-old boy was tested using computerized neurocognitive testing-NeuroTrax. During the patient's first testing session before NFB, he scored 72.4 points overall (Global Cognitive Score-GCS), reflecting a below average score in every area except for verbal functioning. Each time the patient came with his mother for NFB, they were first asked if any progress had been made in his behavior/school performance; their response was recorded as a subjective response.

After only 12 sessions of NFB, his NeuroTrax GCS rose to 80.1 points overall. His memory score increased from 58.1 to 76.7, executive functioning from 49.1 to 74, and attention from 31.6 to 62.7. His family could see improvements with his vocabulary and overall functioning. He was tested again after another 18 sessions (total 30 sessions) scoring 85 points (GCS) on Neurotrax, and then another time after an additional 30 sessions. After 60 NFB sessions, his GCS rose to 94.1 points on neurocognitive testing. The patient's memory score was now 85.1, his executive functioning had reached 91.2 points, and his attention scored 86. His information processing speed (previously too low to score) now achieved 73.9 points, and his visual spatial score was above average at 118.6 points. In addition to marked improvement on the neurocognitive testing, academic performance in school had also accelerated.

QEEG testing before Z-score LORETA NFB showed marked increase in frontal and central beta power (Figure 4 B). LORETA revealed an area of electrical dysregulation in the anterior cingulate (AC) gyrus (Figure 4 A). Subsequent NFB sessions led to gradual improvement of the patient's school performance. After 12 sessions of therapy, QEEG findings indicated marked improvement of excessive beta activity. Further NFB therapy accomplished an even greater reduction of beta activity (Figure 5 A and B), and reduction of cingulate electrical dysregulation. However, some intermittent intersession fluctuation of beta power was also visible during the course of the treatment.

Case 5

23 year old male was diagnosed with low functioning autistic spectrum disorder characterized as major cognitive dysfunction with aphasia and social interaction problems. In addition, frequent generalized seizures were reported despite valproic acid administration. EEG was read as normal. QEEG showed increase in frontal theta and beta power (Figure 6). After course of LORETA Z-score NFB, seizures completely subsided (for more than 22 months), and an improvement in social functioning was noted. Repeated QEEG also showed an improvement of previously overexpressed beta power (Figure 7).

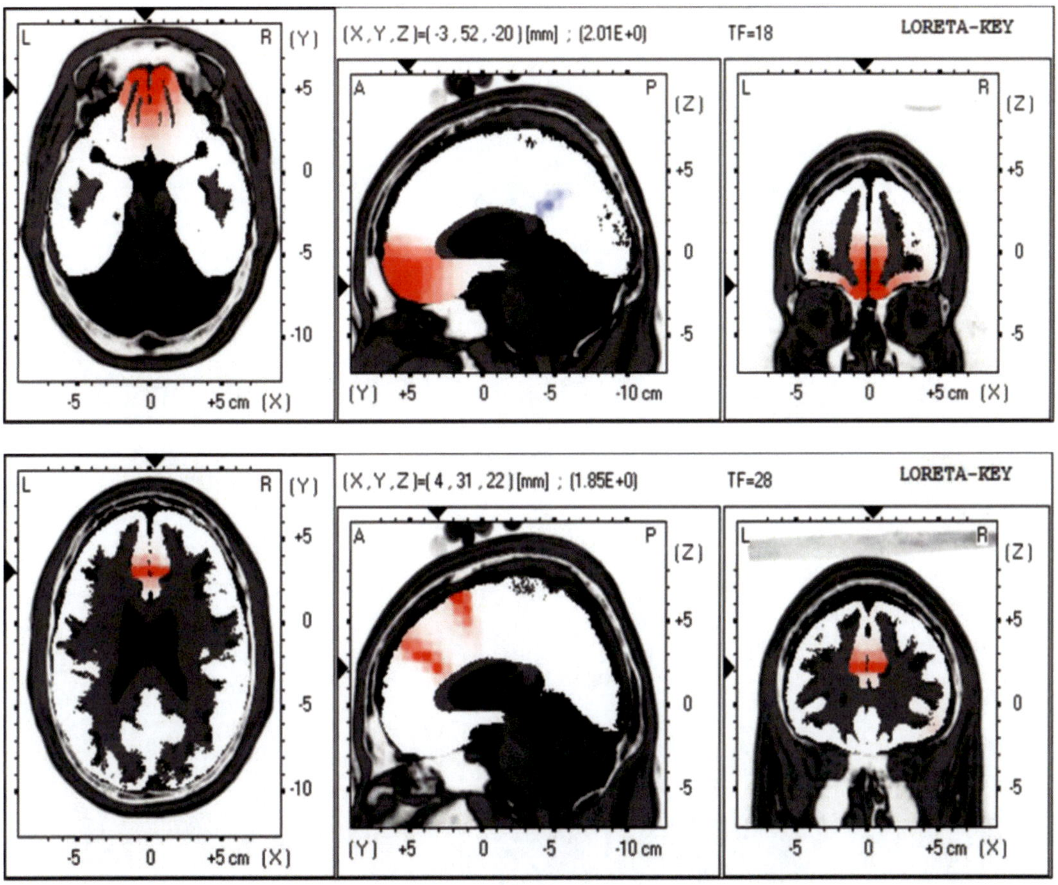

Figure 4 A. 8 year old boy with AS-Pre-NFB-LORETA showed electrical dysregulation of anterior cingulate gyrus-(Brodmann's Area 32 and 24) in beta frequency.

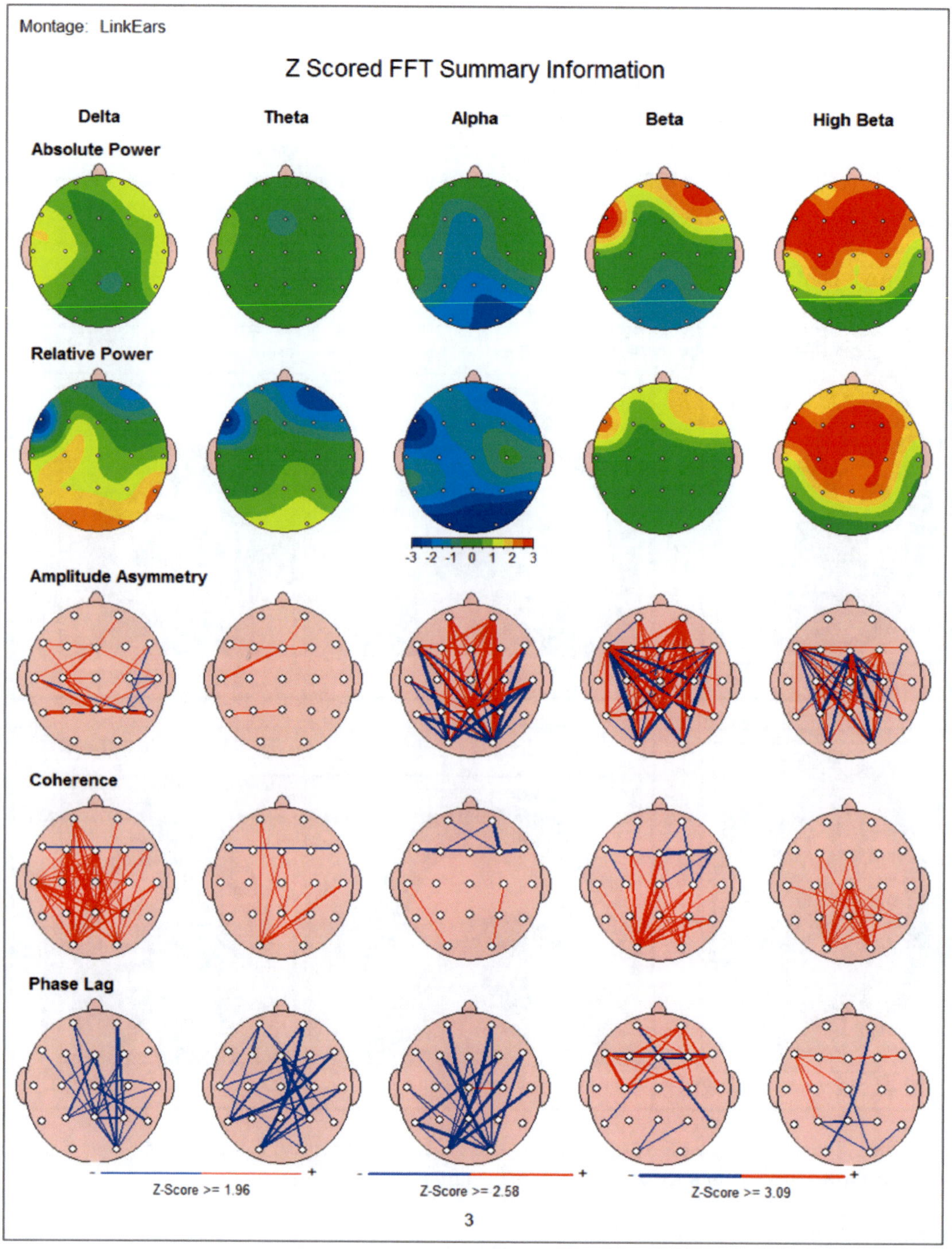

Figure 4 B. 8 year old boy with AS-QEEG before NFB initiation. Noticeable prominent excess of frontal beta and high beta activity depicted in red color. Green color shows brain power within 1 standard deviation, yellow color within 2 standard deviations.

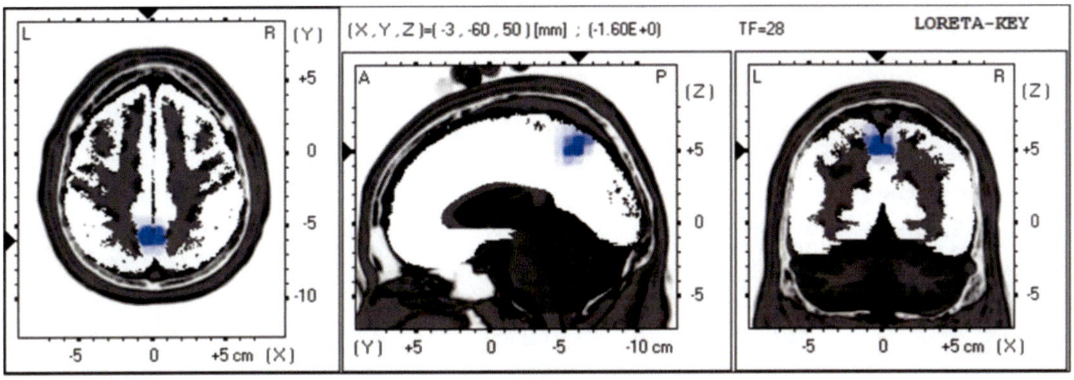

Figure 5 A. 8 year old boy with AS-After 30 sessions of NFB, LORETA no longer shows evidence of anterior cingulate electrical dysregulation.

Case 6

18 year old male who was diagnosed with Asperger Syndrome associated with frequent partial complex seizures. EEG was read as normal on multiple occasions. MRI of brain was also normal. QEEG showed frontal and central increase in beta power. Since this patient did not respond to multiple medications for seizures, in addition to medications, Z-score NFB therapy was initiated. NFB treatment contributed to seizure frequency reduction and improvement in his cognition; however seizures were not completely eradicated. So far this patient completed 51 sessions of NFB over the period of 18 months.

Case 7

14 year old female with Asperger Syndrome (manifesting mostly as behavioral problems with no major cognitive problems) initiated NFB therapy on request of her mother. Her cognitive testing was WNL with GCS-100.8. Her QEEG showed increase in frontal and central beta power. After completion of 7 NFB therapy her mother indicated some improvement in her behavior but no major change in brain maps was noted. Her NFB sessions were stopped due to her insurance termination.

Case 8

This is 12 year old boy with autism who initiated NFB therapy and was able to complete eight session of treatment. His exam showed reduced speech output and had problems with following complex commands. His cognitive testing Neurotrax showed low cognitive score including memory-25 and verbal function-25. QEEG revealed high frontal beta power. After 5 NFB sessions, patient's mother noted some positive behavioral changes and improved speech output was noted. In addition, follow up brain maps indicated some reduction of excessive frontal beta activity. Patient was subsequently lost in follow up.

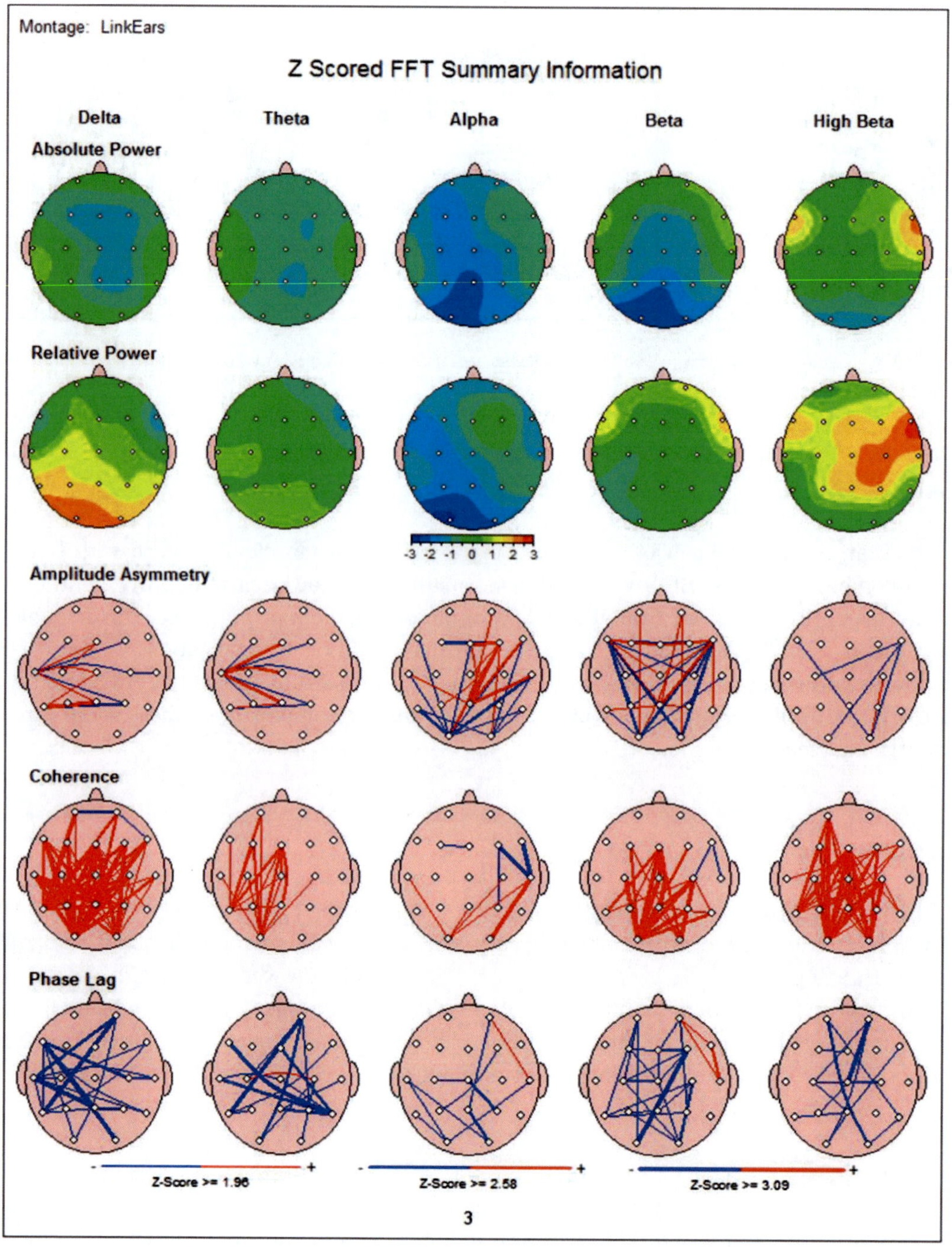

Figure 5 B. 8 year old boy with AS-QEEG after 30 sessions of NFB. Major reduction of frontal beta and high beta activity is noted (reduction of red).

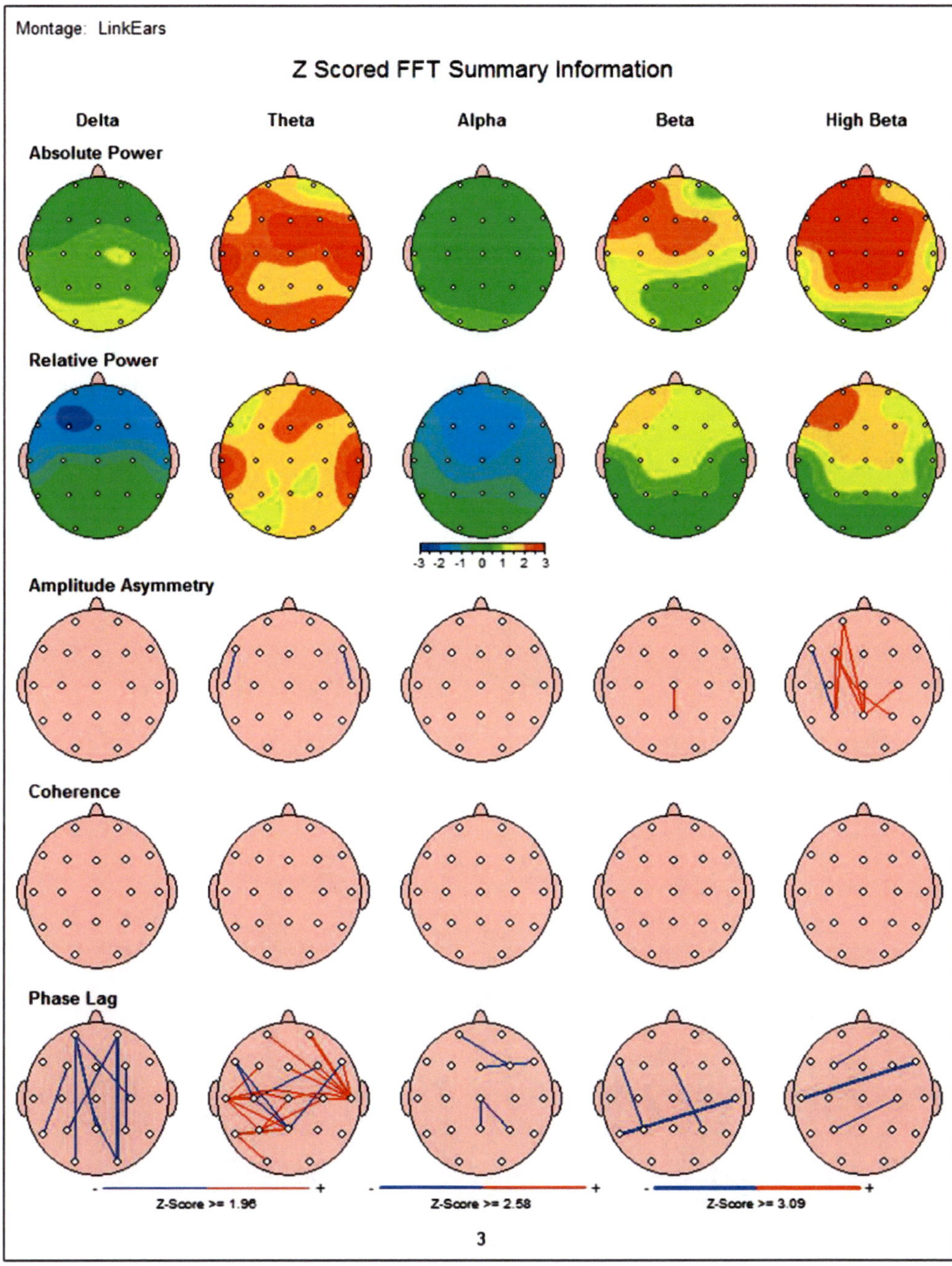

Figure 6. QEEG of 23 year old autistic male-before completion of NFB. Markedly increased frontal beta power was recorded, as well as frontal and temporal theta power.

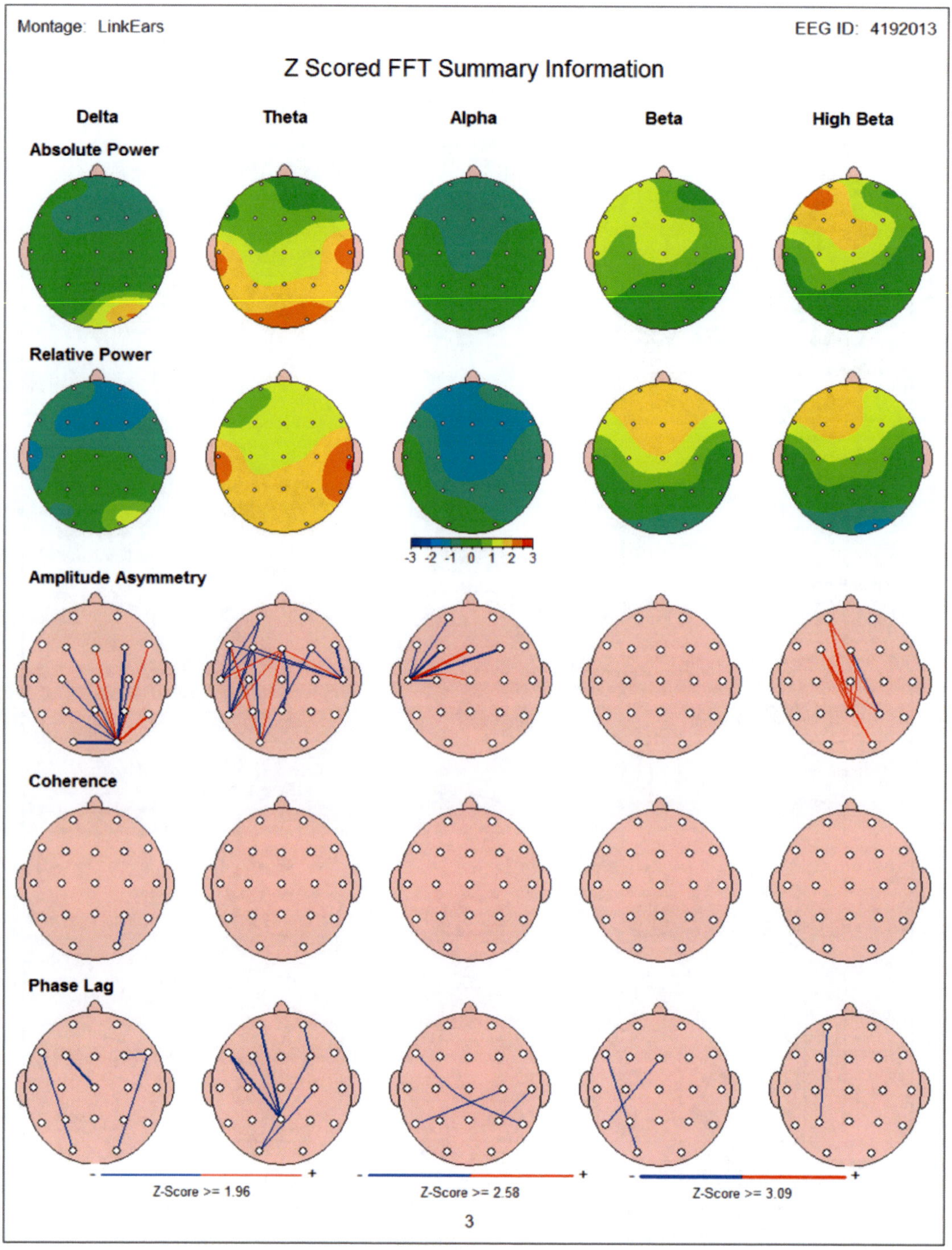

Figure 7. 23 year old autistic male-QEEG after completion of the course of NFB-marked reduction of previously overexpressed beta and theta power is noted.

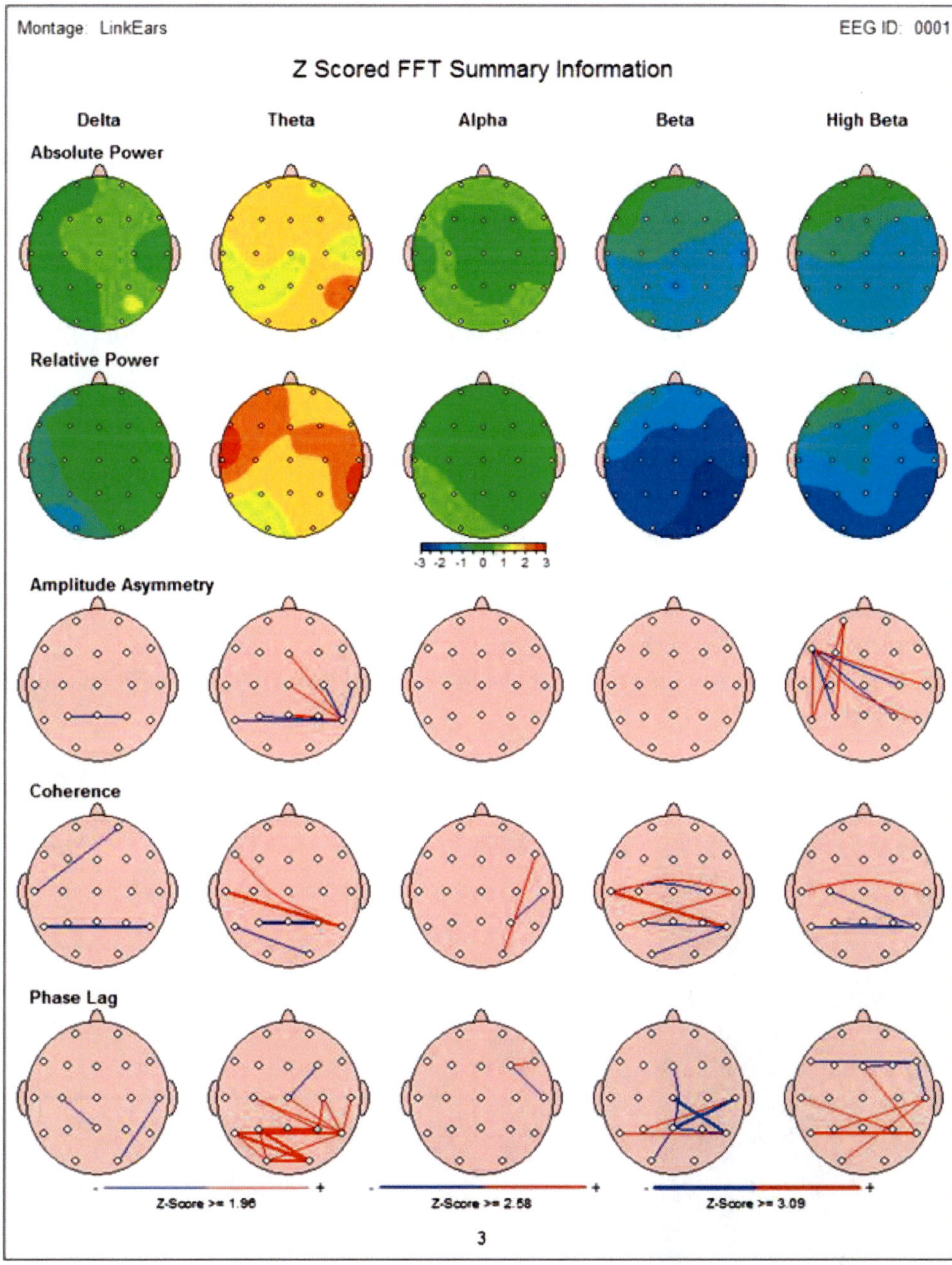

Figure 8. QEEG of 18 year old student with AS with noticeable increase in frontal and temporal theta power.

Case 9

This is 18-year-old male student who presented for an initial evaluation with his mother. His mother reported that he had problems with focusing, concentration and speech expressive functions. In addition, social interaction problems were reported, including a difficulty in making friends and generalized clumsiness. He was not taking any medications. He was a freshman at a local university with very good performance in mathematics and physics (A) - however poorer performance in English and philosophy (B, C). His examination showed monotone type of speech with decreased speech output and reduced facial expression. Some reduction of fine motor movements was also noted during the exam. Initial workup was unremarkable except QEEG, which showed increased theta activity in the frontal and temporal (Figure 8) region.

The patient and his mother were not interested in medication therapy.

Subsequent computerized neuropsychological testing (Neurotrax) showed evidence of major verbal deficiency (see Figure 9). The global cognitive score was below expected (93.2) and most deficient for verbal function (35.5).

Since Z-score LORETA NFB became available in our office, the decision was made to initiate this treatment modality in order to see whether his speech expressive dysfunction could be corrected. A total of 10 sessions of combined surface and LORETA Z-score NFB was completed, and then another computerized neuropsychological testing was conducted (Figure 9). A major improvement of verbal function was noted (104.1) with an increase in global cognitive score (103.1).

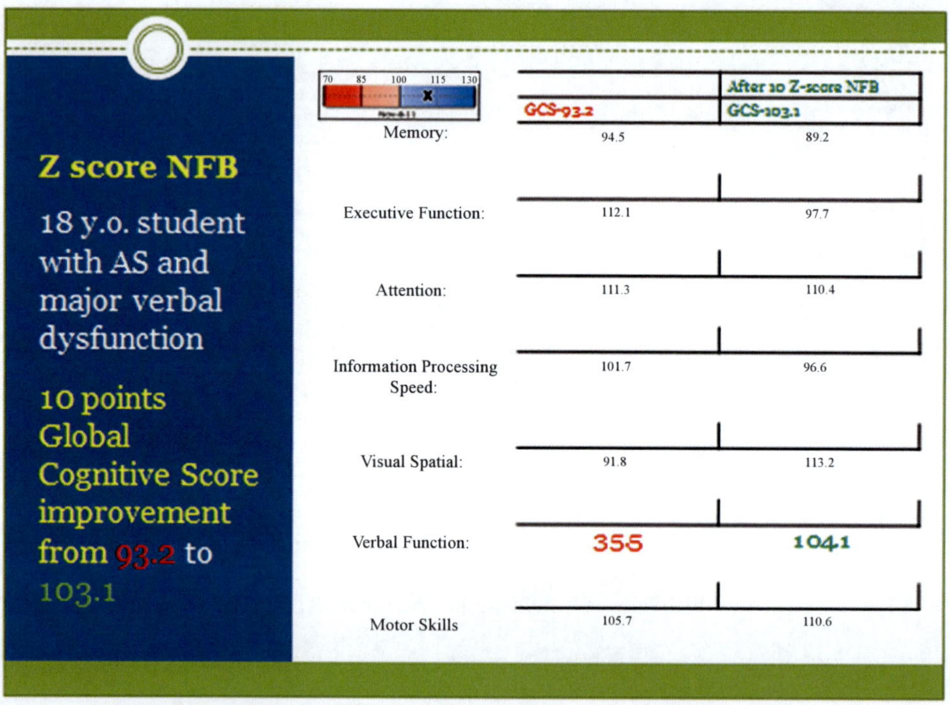

Figure 9. 18 year old male with AS-comparison of computerized neuropsychological testing before and after Z-score LORETA NFB. Left column shows results before NFB, right column after NFB.

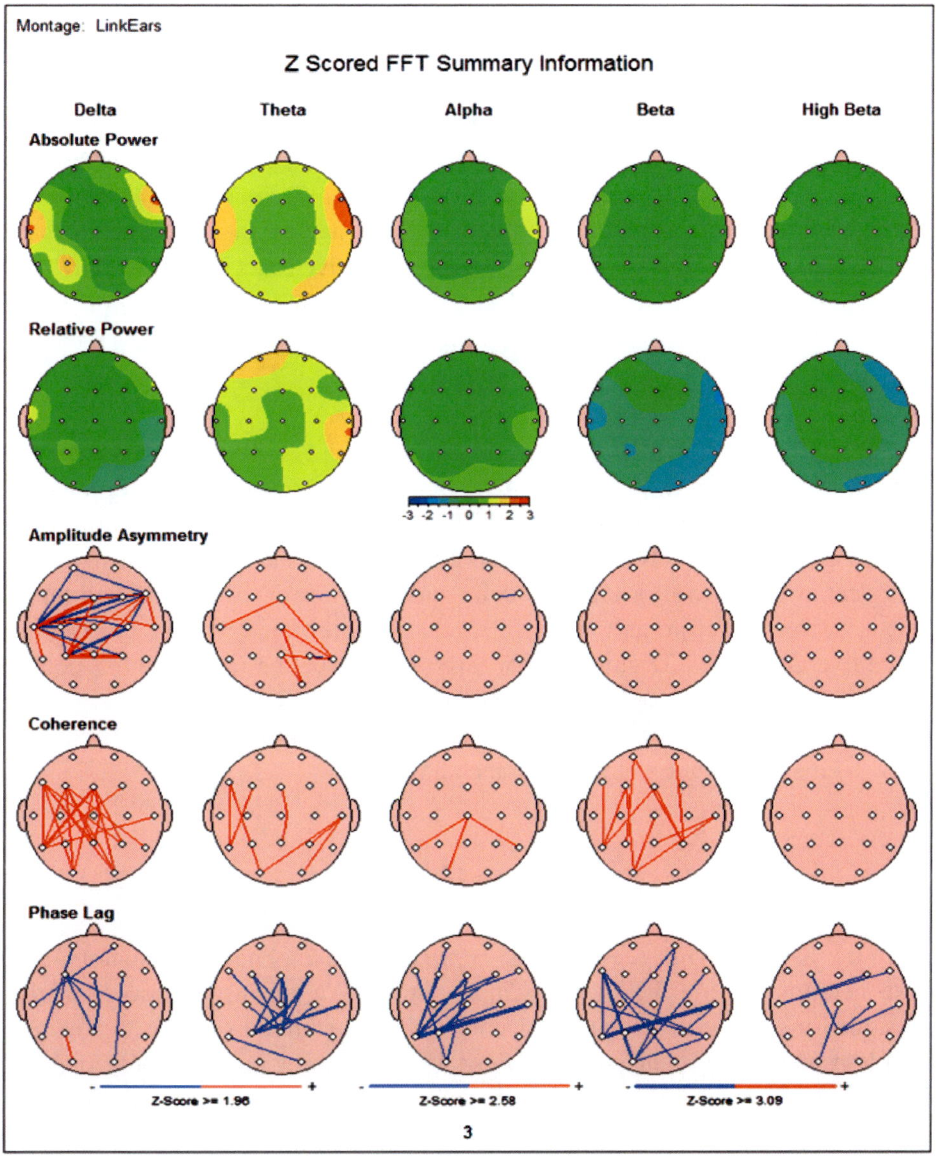

Figure 10. 18 year old male with AS-QEEG after completion of 10 sessions of Z-score LORETA NFB - noticeable reduction of theta temporal power (compared to the initial QEEG recording).

At the same time after Z-score LORETA NFB therapy completion, follow up QEEG was also recorded (Figure 10), which showed a marked reduction of previously overexpressed delta and theta activity.

Subsequently, this patient also reported a marked improvement in university performance, receiving an "A" score in both English and philosophy.

Case 10

This is 14 year old boy with long standing history of behavioral problems who was diagnosed with AS. His MRI of the brain showed mild nonspecific white matter changes. Initial cognitive testing showed no major abnormalities with GCS-94.8. His QEEG before NFB initiation showed an increase in frontal and central beta power. Over the period of 2 years, he has completed 35 sessions of NFB with mild improvement of his behavior. Repeated QEEG showed resolution of previously identified elevated beta activity. Follow up Neurotrax testing showed marked improvement of cognitive function-GCS-105.7.

Discussion

As we can see from the above case reviews, LORETA Z-Score NFB seems to be an effective clinical modality in therapy of ASD. All of the discussed cases reported subjective improvement of their symptoms. In addition, the majority (9 out of 10) of patients were noted to have at least some corrections of QEEG abnormalities, manifesting mostly as increased frontal or central beta power or elevated delta and theta power. In addition, all three patients tested with Neurotrax before and after NFB therapy were found to have marked increase in their cognitive functions. Despite some early on subjective evidence of cognitive and behavioral improvement, a majority of ASD patients required more than 10 sessions in order to fully benefit from neurotherapy. Unfortunately, some of our patients were able to complete only a few NFB sessions due to their insurance limitations.

Conclusion

LORETA Z-score NFB seems to be a very promising neuromodulatory therapy for variety of neuropsychiatric disorders, including ASD. We are in the process of receiving a grant designed to further investigate efficiency of this technology in the treatment of ASD. After implementation, we will be able to enroll much larger numbers of patients, with the possibility of creating a sham control group that will not be subjected to real NFB therapy.

References

American Medical Association. (2000). Diagnostic and Statistical Manual of Mental Disorders. 4th Edition, Washington, DC.

Coben, R. & McKeon, K. (2009). EEG assessment and treatment for autism spectrum disorders. *Autism File*, *32*, 40–7.

Coben, R. & McKeon, K. (2009). EEG assessment and treatment of seizures in children with autism spectrum disorder: a case example. *Neuroconnections*, 17–2.

Coben, R., Linden, M. & Myers, T. E. (2010). Neurofeedback for autistic spectrum disorder: a review of the literature. *Appl Psychophysiol Biofeedback*, *35*, 83–105.

Coben, R., Mohammad-Rezazadeh, I. & Cannon, R. L. (2014). Using quantitative and analytic EEG methods in the understanding of connectivity in autism spectrum disorders: a theory of mixed over- and under-connectivity. *Front Hum Neurosci.*, *26*, 8:45.

Frye RE, Rossignol D, Casanova MF, Brown GL, Martin V, Edelson S, Coben R, Lewine J, Slattery JC, Lau C, Hardy P, Fatemi SH, Folsom TD, Macfabe D, Adams JB. A review of traditional and novel treatments for seizures in autism spectrum disorder: findings from a systematic review and expert panel. Front Public Health. 2013 Sep 13;1:31. doi: 10.3389/fpubh.2013.00031. Review.

Ghaziri, J., Tucholka, A., Larue, V., Blanchette-Sylvestre, M., Reyburn, G., Gilbert, G., Lévesque, J., & Beauregard, M. (2013). Neurofeedback Training Induces Changes in White and Gray Matter. Clin EEG Neurosci published online.

Jarusiewicz, B. (2003). Efficacy of neurofeedback for children in the autistic spectrum: A pilot study. *Applied Psychophysiology and Biofeedback*, *28*, 311.

Koberda J. L., Koberda, P., Bienkiewicz, A., Moses, A. & Koberda, L. (2013). Pain Management Using 19-Electrode Z-Score LORETA Neurofeedback. *J. of Neurotherapy*, *17*, 179-190.

Koberda, J. L., Moses, A., Koberda, P. & Koberda, L. (2013). Clinical advantages of quantitative electroencephalogram (QEEG)-electrical neuroimaging application in general neurology practice-Clin. *EEG Neurosci.* Oct; *44*(4), 273-85.

Kouijzer, M. E., van Schie, H. T., Gerrits, B. J., Buitelaar, J. K. & de Moor, J. M. (2013). Is EEG-biofeedback an effective treatment in autism spectrum disorders? A randomized controlled trial. *Appl Psychophysiol Biofeedback.* Mar; 38(1),17-28.

Lilienfeld, S. O. (2005). Scientifically unsupported and supported interventions for childhood psychopathology: A summary. *Pediatrics*, *115*, 761–764.

Logothetis, N. K., Pauls, J., Augath, M., Trinath, T. & Oeltermann, A. (2001). Neurophysiological investigation of the basis of the fMRI signal. *Nature*. *412*(6843),150–157.

Lubar, J. F. (1997). Neocortical dynamics: Implications for understanding the role of neurofeedback and related techniques for the enhancement of attention. *Applied Psychophysiology and Biofeedback*, *22*, 111–126.

Oberman, L. M., Hubbard, E. M., McCleery, J. P., Altschuler, E. L., Ramachandran, V. S. & Pineda, J. A. (2005). EEG evidence for mirror neuron dysfunction in autism spectrum disorders. *Cognitive Brain Research*, *24*(2), 190–198.

Pascual-Marqui. R. D., Michel, C. M. & Lehmann, D. (1994). Low resolution electromagnetic tomography: a new method for localizing electrical activity in the brain. *Int. J. Psychophysiol*, *18*(1), 49–65.

Pineda, J. A., Brang, D., Hecht, E., Edwards, L., Carey, S., Bacon, M., Futagaki, C., Suk, D., Toma, J., Birnbaum, C. & Rork, A. (2008). Positive behavioral and electrophysiological changes following neurofeedback training in children with autism. *Research in Autism Spectrum Disorders*, *2*, 557–581.

Pizzagalli, D., Pascual-Marqui, R. D., Nitschke, J. B., Oakes, T. R., Larson, C. L., Abercrombie, H. C., Schaefer, S. M., Koger, J. V., Benca, R. M., Davidson, R. J. (2001). Anterior cingulate activity as a predictor of degree of treatment response in major depression: evidence from brain electrical tomography analysis. *Am. J. Psychiatry*. *158*(3), 405–415.

Pop-Jordanova, N., Zorcec, T., Demerdzieva, A., Gucev, Z. (2010). QEEG characteristics and spectrum weighted frequency for children diagnosed as autistic spectrum disorder. *Nonlinear Biomed Phys. 30*, 4(1), 4.

Sansa, G., Carlson, C., Doyle, W., Weiner, H. L., Bluvstein, J., Barr, W. et al. (2011). Medically refractory epilepsy in autism. *Epilepsia*, *52*, 1071–5. doi:10.1111/j.1528-1167.2011.03069.

Shmuel A, Augath M, Oeltermann A, Logothetis NK. Negative functional MRI response correlates with decreases in neuronal activity in monkey visual area V1. Nat Neurosci. 2006 Apr;9(4):569-77. Epub 2006 Mar 19.

Sichel, A. G. (1995). Positive outcome with neurofeedback treatment in a case of mild autism. *Journal of Neurotherapy*, *1*(1), 60–64.

Sitaram, R., Caria, A., Veit, R., Gaber, T., Rota, G., Kuebler, A., Birbaumer, N. (2007). FMRI brain-computer interface: a tool for neuroscientific research and treatment. *Comput. Intell. Neurosci.* 2007:25487. doi: 10.1155/2007/25487.

Sterman, M. B. (2000). Basic concepts and clinical findings in the treatment of seizure disorders with EEG operant conditioning. *Clin Electroencephalogr*, 31, 45–55.

Tan, G., Thornby, J., Hammond, D. C., Strehl, U., Canady, B., Arnemann, K. et al. (2009) Meta-analysis of EEG biofeedback in treating epilepsy. *Clin EEG Neurosci*, *40*, 173–9.

Thatcher, R. W. (2012). Handbook of QEEG and EEG Biofeedback. Electronic edition.

Thatcher, R. W. (2013). Latest developments in live z-score training: Symptom checklist, phase reset, and LORETA z-score biofeedback. *Journal of Neurotherapy*, *17*, 69–87.

Thompson, L. 1., Thompson, M., Reid, A. (2010). Neurofeedback outcomes in clients with Asperger's Syndrome. *Appl Psychophysiol Biofeedback*, *35*(1), 63-81

Viscidi, E. W., Triche, E. W., Pescosolido, M. F., McLean, R. L., Joseph, R. M., Spence, S. J. et al. (2013). Clinical characteristics of children with autism spectrum disorder and co-occurring epilepsy. *PLoS One*, (2013) *8*, e67797. doi:10.1371/journal.pone.0067797

Young, K. D., Zotev, V., Phillips, R., Misaki, M., Yuan, H., Drevets, W. C. & Bodurka, J. (2014). Real-time FMRI neurofeedback training of amygdala activity in patients with major depressive disorder. *PLoS One*. 2014 Feb 11, 9(2):e88785. doi: 10.1371/journal.pone.0088785. eCollection 2014.

Zumsteg, D., Friedman, A., Wieser, H. G. & Wennberg, R. A. (2006). Propagation of interictal discharges in temporal lobe epilepsy: Correlation of spatiotemporal mapping with intracranial foramen ovale electrode recordings. *Clinical Neurophysiology*. *117*(12), 2615–2626.

In: Asperger Syndrome
Editor: Michael F. Shaughnessy
ISBN: 978-1-63463-810-4

Chapter 6

Re-thinking Evaluation and Treatment in Asperger's Syndrome

Adam Blatner, MD
Texas A&M Health Science Center's
(Round Rock Division) Department of Psychiatry, TX, US

Abstract

I hope to offer some tools for thinking more clearly about the needs of people diagnosed with this condition. The goal is work positively with their various strengths and weaknesses so as to promote morale and to encourage them. Clinicians should address the family, too, in the same way. It's not a question of the disorder itself that these people have, but rather getting to know and effectively help the person who happens to "have" the disorder or some behavioral, social or other difficulties.

Keywords: Asperger's, counseling and psychotherapy

Introduction

Asperger's Syndrome, sometimes called Asperger's Disorder, is also now classified by the American Psychiatric Association's latest 5th edition of the Diagnostic and Statistical Manual (DSM) as part of the category called Autistic Spectrum Disorder. I will use the abbreviation AS to refer to all the terminology, and also note that some few—including myself—simply refer to these people as having a "social learning disability." Although there are a variety of sub-disabilities, heightened sensitivities, and other elements that appear to various degrees, the realm of social relations seems to be most prominent. People with AS have difficulty in noticing or responding appropriately to subtle interpersonal cues, or expressing the kinds of social cues that most people take for granted.

Howard Gardner (1993) noted that people have a number of types of intelligence, and some people are quite good in one way, within the mainstream in other ways, and occasionally rather poor in one or another domain—and AS represents poor function in the domain of "interpersonal intelligence." In spite of this, one of the points to be made in this chapter is that with accurate assessments of strengths as well as weaknesses, most can be helped to live more satisfying and productive lives.

I'm a child and adult psychiatrist with over 40 years of experience. Some children have been referred for symptoms of AS. They may be being called names such as "dork" or "geek" by peers, or having difficulties with parents who don't know how to work with them. This operates on a spectrum: Some kids have severe difficulties, while others are only slightly noticeable. Teachers, special education teachers, school psychologists, counselors, child and adult psychiatrists, and other mental health workers are not infrequently presented with individuals who may have been given other diagnoses. I hope this article will offer some general perspectives that supplement the other chapters in this book.

Indeed, sometimes what's a weakness in one area—e.g., social relations—ends up being part of their talent: These folks are less concerned about social interactions and can therefore concentrate on impersonal tasks. It's important to be able to think about how one's makeup might be a gift in certain circumstances. For example, some people with AS are adept at discovering glitches in computer programs, and some businesses have expressly hired "aspies" (as some with AS have taken to calling themselves) for this ability! These folks, gathered together, sometimes feel a little sad for "neurotypicals"—a term people with AS use to note those who cannot do these more focused tasks.

Naming the Problem

The word root of "diagnosis" means something like "seeing through." Making a "good" diagnosis means not merely giving a disorder a label, but rather taking into account the whole person who has the disorder. There's an assessment of other strengths and weaknesses, and this more holistic process is what is needed.

For some who have heard the terms, either Asperger's Syndrome or Autistic Spectrum Disorder, the names offered may have unknown connotations. That is to say, the meaning of these terms may be perceived as either liberating or damning. So much depends on how the words are used—note: They are just labels! Their meanings are shifting and context-dependent!

Diagnostic labels, though problematic in some ways, are useful in some school systems as ways of gaining access to certain services. Does the subject qualify? A label makes a difference. They're not useful if families or the person himself uses the label to feel bad about himself, as a stigma. It's true that people with AS may never make for great salespeople, for example, but there are many jobs and some kinds of social settings where they can have a place and be happy!

Help the child and the family to find and use the words that best describe their problem. Beware of imposing labels that may have emotional impacts that you don't anticipate. Medical diagnoses may be taken as excuses not to try, or that one is literally cursed. Which labels do they hate and why? Help them say, "that doesn't describe me," and then announce what words they want to have used that would be more helpful. This is important. Many people may not say it, but certain labels are felt to demean and/or hurt them. Find out and help them say out loud what words seem more stigmatizing.

This is even more important as an element in evaluation for youngsters with AS in middle school or beyond. Perhaps a phrase such as "I'm not too good socially—it's hard for me to pick up signals or communicate clearly" can be used as a way to ask for help. Meanwhile, some line such as "Well, everyone's good at some things and not others" can be fostered as a kind of encouraging self-talk.

In some ways, perhaps it might be better that AS or should not be considered an "illness" any more than nearsightedness is an illness. For purposes of getting remedial treatment in school, okay. In this sense, AS is noted that a diagnosable entity and in this way falls into what sociologists call a "sick role." Only children with diagnosable entities are considered for special treatment, compensatory education, or some other type of social rehabilitative programs. Many parents are grateful for this side-benefit, and if what's required is that the kid is pasted with a label as "high functioning autism," so be it. However, it must be noted that later in life, though, many of the people so "diagnosed" find a relatively normal and rather satisfying vocation and social life.

So, we should not believe that any label such as AS offers much in the way of guidance. Some family members will be reassured, others shocked or offended. Some have done a fair amount of reading on the internet, others are naive. I think the diagnosis of AS should alert the professional that the person being referred to—child, teenager, or adult—has difficulty in subtle ways—and often they seem distinctly odd, so it's not so subtle—but what they have in common is that these difficulties refer mainly to interpersonal skills, and secondarily to unusual sensitivities.

Diagnosing Co-Morbidities

Note that on occasion children are misdiagnosed as AS when instead—or also—they have other treatable medical problems for which, with a careful evaluation, may be relieved by wearing corrective lenses (i.e., glasses) or hearing aids. Don't assume that these deficiencies have been picked up before! Other physical problems might also account for certain symptoms—anemia, thyroid problems, and so forth.

What is being addressed here is that many people who have a more observable problem may have one or more other problems, too. This is called "co-morbidity." As a more obvious example, a fall can result in both a cut on the scalp and a sprained ankle—two different conditions, both needing attention, but not the same treatment. So it may be with AS: Some kids have this social learning disability compounded by other medical or psychiatric conditions. But those conditions merit diagnosis and treatment also. The predominance of one syndrome does not rule out the complicating presence of other problems.

These can be attitudinal or psychiatric. A common co-morbidity with AS is a pattern of negativity, an "oppositional-defiant disorder," or a "passive aggressive disorder." This simply means that the children have felt misunderstood for some years (and may well have been!) and in response, not having the verbal skills to correct the interpersonal tension, developed a deep pattern of feeling unfairly mistreated and becoming negative or oppositional. It all reflects the point I'm emphasizing that people are complex and cannot be appreciated fully with a single label.

Temperament also complicates the presentation of a person's problem. For example, along with a person's being handicapped with social insensitivity, s/he may also be either very shy or quite bold. The person with AS may be easily hurt and humiliated, or, thick-skinned, seemingly indifferent to subtle put-downs, or teasing. Other possibilities: In spite of being somewhat socially clueless, some people with mild AS are in fact hungry for feeling socially connected, while others seem not to notice or care. Some are very bright in some ways, some not. So, my point in this chapter is to note the various aspects that make each client different.

De-Mystifying AS

As noted at the outset, everybody's got strengths and weaknesses. People with AS may be students or patients or adults in career counseling; they can be any age. In the last several decades increasing numbers of people with low social skills are being diagnosed with this social learning disability. Sometimes it's mild, and sometimes it's overlooked because people have trouble imagining that someone who may be quite bright in many ways can be relatively insensitive in others.

Other people have other things that come hard to them. Some can't carry a tune: Should we call these folks "musical learning disability"? The condition of specific reading or writing disabilities are now commonly recognized. Indeed, it seems that almost everyone has some things that they're terrible at, even though they shine in other areas. So, AS in itself should not be considered a problem, though many with that condition are not well adjusted. It's reasonable to help them to become more adjusted while not fully skilled at socializing. That is to say, not everything about their disability can be fully corrected. It is also so that many with AS can be helped to better compensate for their areas of weakness by (1) building on what talents they have, thus helping them to compensate; and (2) offer some remedial education that minimizes the less adaptive dimensions of their condition.

Considering the Important Variables

Social sensitivity is a spectrum that runs from low to high. On the low end, one is socially "out of it." On the high end of this spectrum—people with what might seen as sort of the opposite of AS, one is naturally talented in roles of host or social organizer. Politicians, successful sales people, some business executives, tend to be good at instinctively reading people and social situations and responding effectively to them. There are people who are rather good at social togetherness. Most of us are in the middle. On the lower end of the spectrum just described are those with what might be called social learning disabilities. Often they are teased or bullied for this social ineptitude. Some are merely introverts, while others have difficulty decoding the kinds of subtle complexities that are unconsciously perceived and correctly responded to by people who have more natural innate interpersonal intelligence.

The degree of social learning disability varies along with many other qualities, such as degrees of wanting friends or not, degrees of intelligence in various ways—or not—and so forth. This point needs to be made repeatedly! The key to helping these people lies in identifying three or four areas of strength and finding ways of putting those skill areas to work in class. For example, if there is a group activity and little Joey is really good at recording machines, let him do the sound recording. Thus he gets to be a part of the team.

It's not as easy to treat as near-sightedness, but other than having a few things in common that qualify a person for this diagnosis, children and adults with Asperger's Syndrome are in other ways quite individual. So recognizing and addressing this individuality is essential.

I've found it useful to identify four elements of individuality: insight, motivation, personal strengths, and family resources. Note that I'm not focusing on the elements of the disorder or weakness per se. Whatever these may be—and these also deserve to be appreciated for what they are—the true meaning of diagnosis is not simply "slapping a label on that which had not been named previously, but a more thorough "through-knowing"—what the Greek word "dia-gnosis" means.

Insight

This is the awareness that they are different, and the challenge is to maintain morale even while recognizing how they are different. We all need to do this in our own way. Still, it sets the stage for any remedial work.

Motivation

This is a complex set of attitudes towards one's own potential for learning, along with feelings towards parents or helping personnel. Are they open to being helped or do they resist it? If the latter, finding out what that resistance is about is key. For example, perhaps previous teachers or parents have been insistent, pushy, scolding, or in other ways overloaded the child. Without being able to articulate why, all these kids can do is push back, be negativistic. It may be difficult to accurately "diagnose" irritability or resistance.

Some kids have been put in an environment pegged too low for their abilities, and they're bored silly. Or they might be put with a bunch of hyperactive kids or be in an otherwise overstimulating environments. Unless such issues are considered, this child will become symptomatic, not as an expression of the underlying social learning disability, but as a result of being exposed to weeks or years of environments that didn't take into account the child's needs.

Some kids get noticed because they are very bright, and the problem is then that they are asked also to respond well to categories that come hard for them. They're quick this way, slow that way. Teachers need to be helped to assess this individuality.

A useful tool is the idea that there's a zone of optimal learning - too slow and the kid gets bored, too fast or remote and the individual gets overloaded (a Russian psychologist named Lev Vygotsky observed this in the early 1930s). The point is to recognize that there is such a range for each skill arena and to structure the learning so that the kid can enjoy some novelty and challenge without going too fast or pushing too hard. This principle really applies to all learning experiences: Some familiarity, but not too much. Some stretch but not overloading. And this varies with each student.

If a kid has had many experiences of gross intrusion, overload, or excessive anger shown to him for what he/she can't help and can't explain, it makes it difficult to engage in a positive learning experience, because he/she brings memories associated with past frustrations to the present. So, counteracting that may be part of the learning—and that's also addressing motivation.

Personal Strengths

There are many of these, but the point to note is that help involves building on strengths and working in compensations for weaknesses. Some weaknesses are relatively fixed and it's best to either drop the effort to develop competence, or delegate the responsibility elsewhere. Some kids are too thin to take up wrestling or too short to do well at basketball. That sort of thing. For nearsightedness, get glasses. I don't know what would apply to AS kids—other than recognizing that there may be certain areas where it's low priority to give attention.

The general idea is to offer a curriculum in which a kid can experience at least 3/4 success. Don't plan remedial experiences in which half the time is spent doing what comes hard or yields mainly frustration. Sustain morale, that's the point. Don't get fixated at what must be learned, but rather support the willingness and ability to tolerate frustration—and for most people, that's about 10 - 20% of learning experience maximum.

Meanwhile, offer other experiences in which the child can gain self-esteem doing things right, sometimes even impressively so. These students need whatever self-esteem they can gain, because the world is letting them know that they are falling short of the mark in so many other ways. So building on the strengths, accentuating the positive, this is key.

Assessing Resources

This is the awkward, but necessary reality that whatever may be done in school can be undone by a family that doesn't understand or isn't "on the same page." Setting up a positive alliance with the family is often difficult, because some parents don't understand. They don't understand not only the special problems of their AS kid, but the general approach of accentuating the positive.

Many people still think that hitting a kid, or speaking harshly (which can have the impact of a hit) is sufficient to correct them—but they don't appreciate that the child has little or no idea of what was done wrong; or if it was wrong, why and how it was wrong; or even if they get that, having any idea how to do it better! This is pretty elementary learning theory, but most people don't get it.

This is because most people—most parents—though seemingly nice—and a few don't even seem nice, because they're angry at the school system or government or whatever and are somewhat defensive—really have little capacity for subtlety. Beneath that proper exterior they are scared, confused, annoyed, sad, and—they feel—unable to admit these vulnerabilities. If it's possible to get parents connected in self-help groups, or to set up such groups, do so! People helping each other can generate more cross-support than reassurance by professionals.

The point here is to get the parents as allies is of inestimable help, and this should be part of any treatment plan. Those parents who are more intelligent, motivated, and informed might be able to be utilized as leaders for such self-help parenting groups, or supported as coaches for the other parents.

Beyond AS

Much of what I'm saying might be applied equally to families with kids who have other kinds of special abilities and/or disabilities—the hard of hearing, vision-impaired, intellectually gifted, those with mobility disorders, etc. The point here is at times to minimize the sense of being all that special with this specific diagnostic category and to recognize that kids with special problems share special needs, and their parents and helpers also share in the need to have their challenges recognized.

Then there's the recognition at another level of what is shared in common by the diagnostic label, and then at a third level the recognition among parents that each child has his or her own unique mixture of sensitivities, strengths and weaknesses. Thus, there are three levels: Parents of special kids need certain supports, encouragement, and education. They need help in sharing and recognizing the challenges of the specific way their kids are special; and then they need support in recognizing how each of their kids are different, in spite of their sharing some common features.

This may seem obvious to some, but know that it is very not obvious to others: Some teachers or their consultants can become so caught up in the esoteric particulars of the AS condition that they overlook the common issues at hand. It's easy to stumble and assume that they are so obvious that they must be taken into account: All too often what seems obvious to some is not at all obvious to others!

Another facet of family resources—other than attention to the education and emotional support for family members—is sheer economics. We should not assume that families can afford many aspects of special care, including, for example, the cost of getting the kid to the school or gym. Transportation is sometimes fraught with complications. Scheduling is a related problem. Lest I be accused of thinking more like a social worker than a psychiatrist, I want to own that thinking like a social worker is often closer to the point of what needs attention. It's a label I honor.

AS has been associated with a more flagrant and odd condition, but with special education expanding for kids with mild emotional difficulties, kids, teens, and even adults and parents who have mild forms of this condition qualify. What's going on is that they don't sense the subtle interpersonal cues, the nonverbal communications, the implications associated with voice tone, the looks and word that others who are more socially integrated absorb both consciously and unconsciously.

Remediation Planning

Notice that I don't talk about "treatment." In other disabilities, the treatment is to correct what can be corrected, say, by wearing glasses or hearing aids. A better term is remediation. Teachers or counselors should attempt to schedule the day so that a youngster with AS has a significant preponderance of success experience. That means that the focus should be on subjects or activities that the kids do reasonably well. Do not over-emphasize remedial work. You may offer some if it's presented as a stretch, but too much will be discouraging. I suspect a ratio of at least three successes to one hard challenge is okay, four successes to one hard challenge even better.

It's demoralizing if they spend more than about a fourth of their time struggling with their weaknesses. Part of the teacher's job, then, is to find what they can tolerate and stretch them a bit. Even for this they need plenty of encouragement. Perhaps peer support from a kid who has a similar problem is possible.

The key is not to be overly impressed with the labels and writings about make-up, catch-up, rehabilitative, etc. If there's too much focus on what's wrong, it's a huge downer. The focus on what comes hard can evoke counter-productive feelings of discouragement. Alfred Adler spoke with clarity about the need to encourage the child. He believed that many people were quite discouraged for various reasons, and the counselor was there to encourage them. The opposite is discouragement, also known as burn-out. Put the morale of the child first. This doesn't mean don't challenge him or her, but don't do it too much. Assessing how much is too much is the job of a creative and sensitive teacher, but should not be second-guessed by an administrator who isn't working closely, watching for signs of overload.

The concept of popularity is also questionable. Some kids develop more social skills and are involved more in what is considered popular. Children or adults with AS tend not to be among them, but may do well in activities that are less popular, and at times even mocked by the more popular youngsters. The point is to help those with AS find a few activities they do like and make the most of this.

Another word that may be misleading is "normal," and it's worthwhile recognizing that many kids who are otherwise normal fall above or below, the average range in some areas. So again the semantics of popular or normal should be questioned. "Normal," after all, merely reflects a statistical norm on some dimension.

Yet nowadays it's useful to identify special talents or disabilities because school systems will accommodate to these if they are noted, diagnosed. It's also good for families to have some terms that they can put in for doing internet searches, to see what other people in the world are doing with these kinds of problems. There are organizations and newsletters.

In other words, whatever the disability, each person deserves an individual diagnosis, not of what's wrong, but equally or more what's right. Is the patient bright or dull and in which way? What limitations and special abilities are present? Temperament, attitude, family support— these kinds of variables make huge differences. The focus then should be only partly on the disorder; more effort should be given to the other variables that are often crucial to the treatment plan, the strategy for collaboration among a variety of parents, professionals, relatives, and friends.

The main thing is that social sensitivity and the learning of the niceties of interaction depends to some degree on innate ability rather than being something anyone can do well.

Some folks pick up on this easily and for others it comes hard. Howard Gardner in the 1980s described several kinds of intelligence, and interpersonal intelligence was one category. Some people are naturally adept at picking up languages, have a feel for mathematics, a knack for fixing things, an innate talent for sports. Similarly, some people are naturally good with people—and for some this is not easy. It's not that this last group are uncaring, but rather that they just don't pick up on the skills that others take for granted.

I prefer to think of this problem as social learning disability. Some folks are naturally good at it, and these make for successful salesmen, politicians, hosts. Most are in-between. For some, the skills involved in interpersonal interchange develop with more difficulty. It is a spectrum.

The "autism" spectrum refers in my mind to those at the bottom third of the total spectrum. These folks in their mildest form were the slightly nerdy kids—pretty healthy in their own world, but not the stars of the school. The bottom third of that bottom third were identified as problematical or autistic. In working with some of these youngsters, I found they varied according to many other variables:

Some were very bright or skilled in other ways—occasionally prodigiously so. While this unusual skill is not present in all youngsters (or adults) with Asperger's, it's worthwhile keeping this dynamic as a possibility. Some people with social learning disability are more interested in being socially accepted than others. That's another variable. The key there is to help them find others who will enjoy their innate abilities and overlook their disabilities.

Summary

The main point then is that kids with any disability need a comprehensive diagnosis that touches not only on the subtle variations that others describe in this book, but more, on the other parts of their personality. What is their attitude? What other strengths do they have? How might helpers build on these?

At home, though labels are ambiguous. Kids of all kinds should be charged with certain chores and their disability should not be an excuse. However, a qualification is needed—and this applies to other kids with other strengths and disabilities. The chores should utilize strengths, work around disabilities. That is, if a kid is good at drawing and making signs, let him do that, but since he has no legs, say, he's not the one to go to the market on errands. This is sensible even for kids without gross disabilities.

Before the middle of the 20th century we expected every child to be good at everything and if they weren't, many mistakenly believed it was because they didn't try hard enough. We now know that to be misleading. Gradually we learned that every kid has some kind of disability, or at least weakness—reading, sports, writing, speaking, etc.—and the same kids often have certain things they do easily—one of the other activities. The illusion that everyone can do everything needed to be dissolved. In its place are more individualized learning programs. Kids who are bright in certain ways need stimulation and lessons adjusted to their ability; those who are slow in other ways need some remediation.

References

Nowadays much can be found on the internet, searching for specifics, self-help groups, information that is more cued into the individual issues relevant to a person's problem. Do a search, starting, perhaps, with: http://en.wikipedia.org/wiki/Asperger_syndrome

Gardner, H. (1983; 1993). *Frames of Mind: The theory of multiple intelligences.* (2nd ed.). New York: Basic Books. http://aspergerspresentation.wikispaces.com/Annotated+Bibliography

Grandin, T. (2014). The way I see it: a personal look at Autism and Asperger's. (3rd edition.) http://www.templegrandin.com/

Steward, R. (16 August, 2014). Lesser-known things about Asperger's Syndrome. http://www.bbc.com/news/blogs-ouch-28746359

In: Asperger Syndrome
Editor: Michael F. Shaughnessy

ISBN: 978-1-63463-810-4

Chapter 7

.... with the end in mind!

Robin A. Wells*
Eastern New Mexico University, NM, US

Abstract

Much information is available regarding Autism Spectrum Disorders, including Asperger Syndrome, and addressing school-aged children. Often missing in the literature is information about adults with Asperger Syndrome or those transitioning from school to the adult world of living and work. This chapter addresses Lessons Learned from work with, and support of, adults with Asperger Syndrome and their families.

Keywords: Autism Spectrum Disorder, Asperger Syndrome, education, and training

Introduction

As many of us are aware, Stephen Covey's *The 7 Habits of Highly Effective People* (2005) states as Habit Two – "Begin with the end in mind." Now while this has application to our personal relationships and our priorities and values, I believe the statement of Habit Two has application to us, as families and educators, as well. Whether our vocational setting is early intervention in the natural environment through transitions into public school settings and then into adulthood, professionals should not just be concerned about the one to three years that a child might be in their care or classroom.

Professionals should be working closely with families in not only providing services and supports to individuals with Asperger Syndrome when they are young and from year to year, but we must also always have "... the end in mind" – adulthood, quality of life, self-determination, interdependence, and independence.

The autism spectrum includes all ages and all levels of skills/abilities of individuals. Characteristics that are demonstrated within this disability are as varied as one's skills and

* Corresponding author: Email: Robin.Wells@enmu.edu.

abilities. Unique talents and creativity are also recognized across the spectrum, and while Asperger Syndrome had been included in the previous Diagnostic and Statistical Manual of Mental Disorders (DSM–IV-TR, 2000), we are now all aware that this specific identification has been excluded from the DSM-5 (2013) edition. Controversy aside (as to whether this condition exists or not; or should have been included in the current edition or not), many families and professionals recognize unique talents, creativity, skills, abilities, and characteristics that are demonstrated by individuals within the spectrum.

The previous definition and/or identified characteristics of individuals with Asperger Syndrome were the following:

> …severe and sustained impairment in social interaction and the development of restricted, repetitive patterns of behavior, interests, and activities. …significant impairment in social, occupational, or other important areas of functioning. …no clinically significant delays or deviance in language acquisition, although more subtle aspects of social communication may be affected. (DSM-IV-TR, 2000, p. 80)

Again, many of us who live and work with individuals with Asperger Syndrome realize that within this category there is a continuum of diverse skills and abilities even for the characteristics cited above.

Hans Asperger (1906-1980) may have been rolling over in his grave as the discussion was being held as to whether this unique group of individuals is indeed outside of the autism spectrum, or truly exist at all. Obvious differences are evident much more now in of our society than in our past history, and these differences in language, cognition, learning, social-emotional well-being, behavior, etc., are more diverse and spread across a continuum with ever-graying lines. The importance of recognizing an individual's unique differences is critical in supporting our fellow members of society in navigating the ever-complex world in which we work, travel, play, and co-exist. This is why we must always have "…the end in mind."

Trusting Relationships

Knowing. Those of us who are in helping professions should never stop acquiring new knowledge and information in the specific field of our discipline, as well as in other disciplines that have implications for our practice. For a professional who earns any type of terminal degree, a life-long journey of learning awaits them. In the 48 years in the educational profession (beginning as a speech/language pathologist for 32 years in the public schools), the new information that has been discovered in how to support individuals along the autism spectrum and with Asperger Syndrome is vast. One could never know everything. What is most important about this field and working with this unique group of individuals is that THEY teach us. All one has to do is be honest and open, allow the individual and the family to know that you are dedicated and committed to learning and growing alongside them, and supporting them in the best way that you can.

Understanding. Continuing that life-long journey of learning has allowed many professionals to better understand the challenges that are present within the individual as well as those challenges outside of the individual. Moving from the perspective/perception of the disorder being caused by a traumatic event and being an emotional/behavioral disorder, to our current understanding of there being neurological differences manifested by multiple factors and having no one single cause is an incredulous learning journey for us all. The challenge for many of us who have been learning and working alongside individuals with this disability and their families is that the majority of professionals in the field of education (and society in general) are still unaware of the insight and information that changes the whole understanding of this disorder and how best to support individuals. I'm waiting for the day when everyone is aware and treats individuals and their families with the respect and dignity that is so deserved.

Conversations

Although the original DSM-IV-TR® (2000) definition indicated that there should be no clinically significant language delay, there are instances where some children have been slow in acquiring language and have unique intonation, rhythm, or pedantic types of speech. Recognizing that speech and language are two distinct components of communication, individuals with Asperger Syndrome may still be in need of supports in the pragmatic and social abilities and use of language.

Theory of mind. The theory of mind is the ability to understand and acknowledge other people's states of mind rather than only perseverating on your own wants, needs, emotions, knowledge, and mental states. This ability enables us to consider another person rather than us being consumed with ourselves, and allows us the ability to realize that not all individuals are thinking in the same way or about the same things as we are. This ability has been identified as an area of needed development in individuals with Asperger Syndrome. Might this be a reason why individuals are unable to interact socially with others, follow another's conversation or interest, or ask additional questions to show that they are following the person's train of thought? Individuals are also thought to have challenges with "reading" body language, facial expressions, and the subtle cues that may be given when another indicates that they would like the interchange to cease. These again are skills that often must be taught through drawing attention to how others are showing us signs that we need to learn to interpret. When around family and friends this may be easily addressed and practiced; as well as having the possibility of addressing this skill in social situations when with supportive peers and adults.

Thinking process. A student, when taking an introductory course in special education, posed a question to the professor while receiving instructor tutorial support privately. The student stated first, "When I was reading about autism and Asperger Syndrome I think that I might have some of the symptoms" and then, "Do you think that I do?" And the professor responded, "Why are you thinking that, what types of 'characteristics' do you think that you might have?" This faculty member had been suspicious that this student indeed had Asperger Syndrome however had not been diagnosed while in high school. A question might be "Would this diagnosis be important now?" Being able to have an ongoing probative conversation over the semester allowed the student to delve into why she reacted to certain situations, her challenges with socially making friends, her anxieties and tentativeness in new situations, and so on. Over the semester the faculty member and the student developed a trusting relationship, with the student demonstrating self-determination in switching her major area of study to that of her strength, recognizing that her challenges in school made her far more empathetic to others who may struggle, and that she indeed was growing in strength and skills that she'd never before been encouraged to develop. Rather than dismissing the student's concern, the instructor encouraged the student to address their personal questions/concerns, allowed nagging questions from previous negative educational experiences to be dissected and reconsidered for their clarity, and supported the student's value towards development.

Self-talk. There may be individuals who believe that the self-talk that often occurs in our heads is really a person speaking to them. This occurrence certainly requires clarification and reassurance. Many individuals may be taught how to problem-solve situations, decrease anxious moments, diffuse mounting feelings of anger, or re-think their perceptions of others' behavior by demonstrating our own thinking processes by voicing them out loud. An individual, who had been bullied not only at school but also in her job at a grocery store after graduation, had the internal belief that people did not like her. She was invited to participate on a United Way Relay for Life team of higher education faculty in her hometown as she was known to walk everywhere in the little city. One faculty member specifically walked with this young lady around the athletic arena and noted that she greeted everyone with "Hi, how are you doing" when she passed them. Many individuals ignored the young lady's friendly overtures, however, some would say, "Hello" or "Hi, Patsy" to her. The young lady would state each time there was no response to her greeting, "They don't like me." The faculty member decided to talk to Patsy about the fact that perhaps people were thinking of other things, people were busy talking with their walking partner, or perhaps they had been paying attention, but that it was okay if they didn't respond. After repeatedly making these comments to Patsy on their laps around the arena, the faculty member began to hear her say after greeting someone with her happy words and welcoming smile with no response, "That's okay, they were probably thinking about other things."

Yes, the desires of individuals along the spectrum are relatively simple. Individuals want to have friends and/or acquaintances, they want to be recognized and acknowledged as being a part of the community, and they want to be respected as a human being and allowed to be who they are. Simple wants and needs – that "sense of belonging" that Maslow (1943) described years ago.

Socializing. Of significant importance to adults with Asperger Syndrome is the ability to socialize if they indeed wish to do that. As discussed earlier, there are many factors that may prevent an individual from having the ability to interact socially with others (language, theory of mind, challenges in reading body language or facial expressions), and there will be additional factors addressed later in this piece that may also make the ability to interact challenging. Early positive, social experiences that may often be facilitated and/or monitored by an adult lay the foundation for future social interactions. Strategizing how to comfortably introduce and involve the individual with Asperger Syndrome into community activities as much as possible, demonstrating appropriate manners, waiting skills and patience, standing in lines, waiting our turn, etc. are invaluable skills best learned when much younger. One of the two most important factors in future employment that has been identified by employers is the ability to get along with co-workers. The start of this skill begins early in a child's development and should be an important goal from birth through five and beyond.

Collaboration

Person-Centered Planning. Although many new ideas and approaches in supporting individuals with Asperger Syndrome have begun due to the advocacy of their families, kudos must also be given to those professionals in the field of disability who are truly committed to the improvement of the lives of the individuals with whom they work and support. A demonstration of this commitment is the development of the Person-Centered Plan. Collaborative conversations among professionals over a period of time (1979-1992) resulted in information, training, materials, and anecdotal accounts of positive outcomes for individuals using this approach (O'Brien & O'Brien, 2000). Groups consisting of supportive group of parents, peers, friends, relatives, and professionals who have the best interests of the individual in mind and who are committed to make hopes/dreams become reality meet consistently in order to gain the individual's perspective, as well as the family's, in how to plan the supports needed to fulfill the person's wishes.

Many other types of collaborative teamwork have created supportive planning groups as well. The McGill Action Planning System (MAPS) provided a more visual way of planning out one's life, hopes, dreams, supports; Essential Life Planning, Circle of Friends, and Getting to Know You introduction booklets also provide insight into what the individual wants rather than what the adults deem to be more appropriate, but oftentimes is much less attractive or interesting to the individual with Asperger Syndrome. After involvement with one of the alternative approaches in reviewing an individual's life, the stale Individual Education Plans (IEPs) that are automatically developed in school systems seem very antiquated and frequently do not achieve the expectations of the vision of life as held by the individual themself.

Quality of Life. There have been five areas identified as providing a *quality of life* for any of us: physical well-being (health, exercise, nutrition), material well-being (work, vocation, income, housing), social well-being (friends, family, relationships), emotional well-being (self-regulation, coping, positive thinking), and development and activity (community activities, museums, cultural activities, leisure activities) (Felce & Perry, 1995). When reflecting about our own individual lives and what makes us feel that our lives are fulfilled, most of these elements are tantamount and needed for our own self-satisfaction. If indeed this is so, do individuals with a disability and/or Asperger Syndrome have the same opportunities, experiences, and exposure to create such a life for themselves? Again, when we begin "...with the end in mind", this should be the ultimate outcome we are pursuring. Our collaborative planning from infancy to adulthood for an individual with Asperger Syndrome should be focusing on providing as many opportunities and strategies for the development of the skills and abilities needed to enhance their life through the relationships and conversations we encourage about their strengths and dreams,.

Burgess and Turkstra (2010) used the Quality of Communication Life Scale (with modifications) to determine perceptions of individuals along the higher end of the autism spectrum regarding their skills/abilities in using social language. As the American Speech-Language-Hearing Association has begun addressing language challenges from a systemic model perspective rather than the previous medical model used, language interventions are implemented more practically in the context and/or environment in which they occur and within personal relationships with other individuals (Burgess & Turkstra, 2010). While perceptions of individuals along the higher end of the spectrum are quite different than peers without ASD, this should not be unexpected. The issue would be, if the individual is comfortable and pleased with where they are, then would this be something that should be addressed. Some might say, "Perhaps individuals do not understand how much fuller and richer their lives would be if their social communication skills were stronger." Excellent point, however, without having established a trusting relationship with an individual, and being able to have in-depth conversations and/or discussions regarding how "neurotypical" individuals perceive social situations, one may not be able to share a different perspective with the individual with Asperger Syndrome. Who is to say that that individual's perception and comfort level are not acceptable? If social behavior or communication skills tend to create more challenges or issues in one's life, or become barriers to obtaining life-long dreams and aspirations, then obviously a trusted family member, professional, or peer must provide positive and supportive strategies to assist the individual in learning new skills. Temple Grandin often states that without the support and interest of individuals who were her supervisors, she would not have known to make changes in her life (i.e., story of supervisor and deodorant). All humans are both independent and interdependent. At several points in our life journeys we need assistance, patience, and understanding from others. Individuals with any type of diverse learning abilities are no different.

Strengths and/or Concerns

Historically the field of special education used a medical model in approaching disabilities. A medical model is one in which disability is viewed as something to be "fixed or cured", and only a specialized group of people are thought to be capable of intervening with this group. This approach also viewed a disability from a deficit model or negative viewpoint, often listing all the weaknesses or deficits on which interventions should be focused. The earlier medical model approach has now been replaced with a strengths-based model. This positive model views individuals with disabilities as part of just being human or being a natural occurrence in all societies. The educational field is urged to use Person First or People First Language, and this commitment was included in the 2004 Reauthorization of the Individuals with Disabilities Education Act. For more information regarding Person First Language, visit the website, www.disabilityisnatural.com, developed by Kathie Snow.

The strengths-based model, or approach, to disabilities is one in which the focus is on increasing the strengths of the individual while acknowledging the concerns, however, goals of the IEP do not just address the identified concerns. When targeting the strengths of an individual, concerns often lessen or decrease, and separate types of supports might be developed specifically for circumventing, minimalizing, or decreasing those areas of concern. Attending to an individual's interests, proclivities, and obsessions may be a clue as to their aspirations or may also be a way to develop strengths more easily.

Positive Behavior Supports. A positive behavior support (PBS) approach to areas of concern focuses on how an individual along the spectrum may be supported in learning new skills; replacing less acceptable behaviors with ones that are as pleasurable, comforting, and functional; teaching coping skills; changing the environment to be more supportive; changing the manner in which adults verbally interact with an individual, and increasing functional language and social skills to name just a few strategies. Parents and professionals also increase their understanding of the underlying causal relationship or link to the demonstrated behaviors, and then a positive plan to support the child in becoming more in tune with their emotions, physical and sensory systems, skills, and interests is developed.

Obsessive-compulsive tendencies. There are individuals with Asperger Syndrome who may also be diagnosed with an additional disorder or neurological condition, and this would be considered a "co-morbid" diagnosis. Many individuals experience obsessive-compulsive tendencies, anxiety, attention deficit hyperactive disorder (ADHD), or sensory integration challenges. Some individuals have been diagnosed with attention deficit hyperactivity disorder when in reality the cause of the high activity level may be a sensory challenge. Not all obsessive-compulsive tendencies should be viewed negatively as many may be turned into a future field of endeavor, vocation, or study for the individual. Templin Grandin has demonstrated that her extreme interests in sensory aspects of calves when being castrated on her aunt's ranch actually spurred her to construct her Squeeze Machine (Grandin, 1986), which she personally used to calm her overanxious physical feelings. Some demonstrations of "being stuck" or obsessed about specific topics of conversation when viewed by others as "inappropriate" have actually been identified by the individual as a means to demonstrate their intelligence to others (Barron & Barron, 2002). "Being stuck" has also been described as a motor movement disorder or inability to volitionally make your body respond in the way you intended (Donnellan & Leary, 1995). The remarkable book written by Donnellan and Leary (1995) provides insight as to why some individuals (even perhaps individuals with Asperger Syndrome) may have difficulty moving away from a topic of interest, a question that may has already been answered, or a detail that has been described to them numerous times. While our understanding and acknowledgment of individuals are vital to our ability to support learning and progress, we must also be aware of perhaps our unconscious reinforcement of obsessions, compulsions, etc. of individuals.

We have been told repeatedly in introductory seminars that individuals along the spectrum often "need" routine and structure in order to avoid tantrums and/or outbursts. If we were to follow this advice, this strategy may be more detrimental than supporting the individual by acknowledging their need for sameness and determining how we might teach individuals how to be more flexible. What we may in actuality be reinforcing or encouraging is rigidity that with the growth and maturity of the individual may morph into the individual's inability to be flexible and "roll with the punches."

Anxiety. Left unaddressed, anxiety may develop into greater social anxieties, a tendency towards isolation, and perhaps a harboring of ill feelings towards peers who may have been bullies or perceived as being mean. Not all individuals experiencing anxiety become overly alert to others and their bullying, however, some individuals may find aggression to be a release for their over-powering anxiousness (Pugliese, White, White, & Ollendick, 2013). Prior to being diagnosed as also having an anxiety disorder, an individual with Asperger Syndrome, with whom this author is familiar, was observed to "self-medicate" to relieve increased feelings of stress. The method of this "self-medication" was that of cutting himself with old-fashioned serrated bottle caps or straight-edged razor blades. While the superficial cuts were not worthy of a trip to the emergency room, they were still very alarming to support staff who had not bothered to inquire as to why the individual was doing this and then linking earlier situations to an anxiety-filled experience. Being with this individual (among so many others), highlighted the importance of having conversations with individuals with Asperger Syndrome to learn of their unique perspectives, perceptions, and feelings. The answers to our puzzlement may be very easily solved with just a wonderful conversation. In this way we may be better able to problem-solve with the individual as to what is needed to diminish stressful situations, acknowledge the situations that cause stress and anxiety, and develop/teach strategies that may be used with ease and confidence.

Sensory issues. The Sensory Profile (Dunn, 1999) is an assessment process used by occupational therapists in determining the "…effect of sensory processing on functional performance in the daily life of a child" (Dunn, 1999, p. 1). Dr. Dunn has made the area of sensory processing her life's research and has, (with the assistance of graduate students) developed profiles for infants/toddlers and for adults. The Sensory Profile has been used to determine differences in individuals with and without autism (Kientz & Dunn, 1997). Interestingly, the Sensory Profile questionnaire does indicate a pattern for those with ADHD; however, the first study with young children with autism did not demonstrate such a pattern much to the surprise of the research assistant raters. While individuals with autism may demonstrate challenges with sensory processing, there was not a distinct profile that was revealed. Within the past few years, however, the Profile was used to study individuals with Asperger Syndrome and the findings seem to indicate that there is a stronger pattern of sensitivities in individuals who are on the higher end of the spectrum. Sensory processing challenges often affect the ability of individuals to participate in everyday activities, learn as other children do, and communicate in ways that develop friendships.

Strategies and Supports

Evidence-based. Educational forces even in early intervention are requiring the use of evidence- or research-based interventions and strategies to be used with any child with a disability. Reasoning for this is to ensure that individuals are receiving quality and proven interventions, strategies, and approaches that have the most reasonable assurance of positive outcomes. Many strategies and positive supports have been proven to be effective for individuals. Some strategies and/or interventions, although not proven effective through research studies, are often implemented or tried by families and/or uninformed professionals. For families, the desire to assist and support their child in any way possible, outweighs the notion of only using those "proven-to-be" strategies, and this is extremely understandable. Some strategies and interventions are easily implemented and without much expense while some "programs" being tried are expensive, extremely structured, and are not always helpful to all individuals.

Folklore. When in graduate school, a professor chastised me for relating anecdotal stories from parents (and from my own experiences) in class regarding strategies or approaches that were being used (unproven and in fact sometime disproved) with great outcomes. The professor referred to these anecdotal tales as "folklore." Anything that was not proven to her through research was determined to be invalid. A lesson learned while working closely with parents is that what works for your child, works for your child. Some proven strategies, etc. may not always be beneficial and should be put aside if tried (obviously in the valid way that the strategy was intended to be implemented) and found to be unsuccessful. Sometimes creative parents and professionals develop the most uniquely individualized strategies that tap into the child's special interests and "whah-la" – success! Personally and professionally I will not disregard "folklore" even though I was publicly embarrassed by the professor, but will rather keep an open-mind to all the possibilities presented.

Concerns. Some concerns that we may have about behaviors demonstrated by individuals may be discarded when the behavior is no longer found to be beneficial. Not all behaviors need to be addressed at once, so we should be very selective when identifying what it is that we feel deserves our attention. For instance, often when language skills are increased through intentional strategies for encouraging interactions, social and play skills increase; therefore, addressing one area of concern often alleviates another area of concern. Intervention provided early and in natural environments typically yields substantive positive outcomes.

Hygiene. As mentioned earlier, there were two important skills identified by employers that an individual needs to have when seeking employment. One was the ability to get along with co-workers, and the second skill needed was good hygiene (which includes bathroom skills). Obviously in our quest for preparing any child for independence, the ability to take care of one's personal hygiene (bathing, grooming, dressing, etc.) also includes the ability to take care of our own bathroom needs AND to be alert to healthy hygiene practices while in the bathroom. In some places of employment there may be only one bathroom for each gender. The expectation would be that an employee would be able to use the bathroom without leaving any residue, and follow the healthy practices of washing and drying hands after using the facility. The earlier that we teach good hygiene practices (and teach the steps needed to be followed), the more quickly this important independent skill may be crossed off the list of life-long skills.

Choices and Self-Determination

Through the years, the field of special education has evolved (hopefully) from prohibiting individuals from doing something unless they were told (allowed) to do so by their teacher. What was created through this previous practice was individuals who were taught to not take initiative, not think for themselves, to always ask for permission, and wait to be told what to do - when to do it - and for how long. Also what previously was a common practice was to provide a tangible (often edible) reward for doing something that was instructed by the teacher. What this created were individuals who depended on being prompted to do something, or acquired what is termed to be "learned helplessness." Educators faulted the individual for waiting or not beginning tasks, when in fact it was the educator who had reinforced the waiting and taught the individual not to respond. A story that provides an interesting example of this is about a group of individuals who were living in "group homes/residences" and were always taken together in a van on community outings. When one of the community excursions was over and the adults were returned to their group residence by the van, the group home supervisor told everyone to get out of the van and go inside. One man was not getting out of the van, so again the supervisor instructed the individual to get out of the van, to which the man said, "What will you give me?" Thus again, the staff or professional had taught this behavior by reinforcing no movement until told or given a reward. From this dilemma came the realization by professionals of the lack of respect for the dignity of individuals, and how in many instances our old ideas and ways of "teaching" individuals was really not supporting long-term growth and independence. Conversations among professionals emerged about how to reverse this negative trend of creating "responders" to instead creating "initiators."

Simple to complex. Early choices of food, toys, play activities, clothes, or what video to watch, and then as children grow older moving to who should we invite to a party, and then to where do you want to live, who might you invite to live with you, or where do you want to work are examples of the path from simple choice or decision-making to the more complex questions facing us when we reach adolescence and adulthood. Pathways to a quality of life in adulthood must be planned and begin when the individual is young. Setting the foundation and groundwork for making simple to complex choices are important elements in providing the individual with Asperger Syndrome the ability to live a fulfilling life. Many of the strategies used in early intervention for choice-making are still relevant in school and community activities. Providing choice using real objects to photographs and words to words only, then reading the words or being able to make verbal choices, link foundational pieces to application in real-world situations. When families and professionals have developed collaborative partnerships, the planning is more easily and seamlessly achieved. The difficult discussions may have already occurred, which then allow the adults to be open and honest with each other in developing workable plans that cross environments and settings with real application.

Allowing and acknowledging. Respect for choices and preferences when children are young are the first steps towards learning self-determination. The ability to speak up for yourself (rather than waiting for someone else's permission to speak or act) and advocating for what you need and want are important lessons to be learned. Providing choices of food from which to select, tasks from which to choose to complete first, or clothes combinations to wear to school are essential elements in learning how to be independent, and asserting one's ability to indicate your individual preferences. As individuals get older, the importance of them being involved in the discussions, the planning, and the development of their own IEPs, are other steps towards independence and self-determination. When included in discussions of strengths, and asked to provide input into what one might like to experience in preparation for their future work setting, the individual with Asperger Syndrome will be able to understand that their opinion counts and that the adults in their world are wanting to support them in their personal goals and dreams. Self-determination also links with the development of a Person-Centered Plan or a McGill Action Plan where the individual is encouraged to express their hopes and dreams, their goals for the future, what they would like to see happen, where they would like to live, and how or what steps are needed in order to achieve their ultimate goal. With "…the end in mind", planning and support in practicing what skills are needed to ensure a future with a positive quality of life is a goal for which to strive.

Hope

Most often what amazes me is how some professionals speak in "absolutes." School psychologists, diagnosticians, learning specialists, and others may be perceived as indicating that the intelligence and skills of the individual being discussed during IFSPs or IEPs is exactly what the results indicate – numbers, skill levels, etc. No one bothers to state that the assessment was completed in one long sitting, with a stranger, in an unfamiliar setting, and without contextual or environmental cues/support provided. Our interpretations of assessment and evaluation information are indicative of a one-time situation only and do not address how the individual demonstrates their intelligence or skills within a natural environment, within the community, or when with familiar people and friends. Those who are skilled in assessment/evaluation may take this into consideration, however, most professionals continue to provide information that the families hear or perceive as "doom and gloom." No one says, "Your child is very young and the possibilities are unimaginable at this time" or "Yes, we may have missed some critical time periods where learning was easier, however, that doesn't mean that your child will not make gains given the right supports and interventions" or "Let's see what will happen when we provide experiences and opportunities to your son/daughter in the community, prepare them for the situation, provide support when in the situation, and talk them through any challenges." Individuals are known to do much better when in typical settings/environments with peers without disabilities. Those of us working with and supporting individuals and their families pre-plan proactively to circumvent distressing situations and/or teach much needed skills and abilities prior to experiencing a potentially stressful situation.

Once after hearing Dr. Tony Attwood speak at an autism conference about his experiences with "Aspies" (the term with which many individuals with Asperger Syndrome refer to themselves), I was able to have him personally autograph his book and have a word with him. I related to him that I had been criticized for being positive with families about the unmet potential of their children and growth, and that an increase of skills/abilities was still possible. Dr. Attwood (personal communication, April 2001) stated, "Never take hope away from parents; it's the only thing that they have." This affirmation of being supportive to families while remaining honest and sincere was empowering.

Conclusion

Strategies that we implement, instructions we give, interactions we have, relationships we build, perceptions we change, realities we acknowledge, skills we strengthen, trust we develop, accomplishments we share, choices we allow, self-determination we encourage, supports we provide, discoveries we make, risks we take, conversations we have, and collaborations we create are all part of our support of others. Professionals begin working with families with infants and toddlers in early intervention programs (Part C), and although we may only spend two short years focused on the little ones, everything that we are doing with families and their children must always keep "…the end in mind." As children move through preschool programs and public school programs, again, we must have "…the end in mind." The years that we spend with children are short compared with the commitment and dedication of the child's family, not to mention the child's whole life itself. A wise professional, Anne Donnellan, once said at the end of a slide presentation at a national autism conference in the 1990s, "Every child, when they are born, should be issued a T-shirt that says – **Don't Waste My Time!**"

For all of us who have the privilege of knowing an individual along the autism spectrum, and perhaps may even have the opportunity to support and develop a trusting partnership with them and their families, the time spent counts! We must make the most of all the time that we are allowed with the individuals and their families we serve – everything matters! So we must always have begin "…with the end in mind."

References

American Psychiatric Association. (2000). *Diagnostic and statistical manual of mental disorders* (DSM-IV-TR®) (4th ed.) (Text Revision). Arlington, VA: American Psychiatric Association.

American Psychiatric Association. (2013). *Diagnostic and statistical manual of mental disorders* (DSM-5™) (5th ed.). Washington, DC: American Psychiatric Association.

Barron, J., & Barron, S. (2002). *There's a boy in here: Emerging from the bonds of autism.* Arlington, TX: Future Horizons, Inc.

Burgess, S., & Turkstra, L. S. (2010). Quality of communication life in adolescents with high-functioning autism and Asperger syndrome: A feasibility study. *Language, Speech, and Hearing Services in Schools, 41*, 474-487.

Covey, S. R. (2005). *The 7 habits of highly effective people.* New York, NY: Simon & Schuster.

Donnellan, A. M., & Leary, M. R. (1995). *Movement differences and diversity in autism/mental retardation: Appreciating and accommodating people with communication challenges.* Madison, WI: DRI Press.

Dunn, W. (1999). *The sensory profile.* New York, NY: Pearson.

Felce, D., & Perry, J. (1995). Quality of life: Its definition and measurement. *Research in Developmental Disabilities, 16*, 51-74.

Grandin, T., & Scariano, M. M. (1986). Emergence. Labeled autistic. Novato, CA: Arena Press.

Kientz, M. A., & Dunn, W. (1997). A comparison of the performance of children with and without autism on the Sensory Profile. *The American Journal of Occupational Therapy, 51*(7), 416-423.

Maslow, A. H. (1943). A theory of human motivation. *Psychological Review, 50*(4), 370-396.

O'Brien, C. L., & O'Brien, J. (2000). *The origins of person-centered planning: A community of practice perspective.* Syracuse, NY: Responsive Systems Associates, Inc.

Pugliese, C. E., White, B. A., White, S. W., & Ollendick, T. H. (2013). Social anxiety predicts aggression in children with ASD: Clinical comparisons with socially anxious and oppositional youth. *Journal of Autism and Developmental Disorders, 43*, 1205-1213. doi 10.1007/s10803-012-1666-x

Snow, K. (2014). *Disability is natural.* San Antonio, TX: BraveHeart Press. Retrieved from www.disabilityisnatural.com

Vandercook, T., York, J., & Forest, J. (1989). The McGill Action Planning System (MAPS): A strategy for building the vision. *Journal of the Association for Persons with Severe Handicaps, 14*(3), 205-215.

In: Asperger Syndrome
Editor: Michael F. Shaughnessy

ISBN: 978-1-63463-810-4

Chapter 8

Neuropsychological Perspectives in Understanding Affective and Cognitive Impariment in Asperger Syndrome: The Case of Facial Expression of Emotions

Maria Elide Vanutelli[1,2], Giovanni Lecci[2] and Michela Balconi[1,2*]
[1]Research Unit in Affective and Social Neuroscience,
Catholic University of Sacred Heart, Milan, Italy
[2]Department of Psychology, Catholic University of Sacred Heart, Milan, Italy

Abstract

The human face is one of the most important stimuli to convey and perceive essential information regarding social interactions, and the capacity to recognize and understand emotions from faces represents a primary social competence, since it supports social communication.

Research has consistently shown that autistic children exhibit inattentiveness and attribute a weak salience and attention to emotional facial expressions, if compared with other non-emotional cues. Moreover, several studies have found that Autistic Spectrum Disorders individuals (ASD) show impaired abilities to decode and understand others' emotions. Nonetheless, the extent of the deficit in facial expression understanding varies within the autistic spectrum.

The intent of the present chapter is to review relevant evidence of facial emotion comprehension in ASD, showing common patterns of impairment within the same clinical spectrum, and to focus on Asperger's Syndrome (AS) behaviors, emphasizing both deficient processes and compensatory strategies. The most important theoretical models on affective and cognitive impairment in autistic and Asperger individuals are discussed, in addition to more recent approaches. They will be described and

* Corresponding author: Michela.Balconi@unicatt.it; Department of Psychology, Catholic University of Sacred Heart, Largo Gemelli, 1.20123, Milan, Italy.

integrated with empirical evidence within a neuroscientific frame, highlighting the neuropsychological perspective as the election level of description in AS study to provide a bridge between the brain and mental functions. The case of facial emotion comprehension is considered as a pivotal example of social behavior, which includes the integration of biological, cognitive and social skills. This approach seems to provide promising advances and suggestions for comprehensive models. Finally, a multi-functional model of facial emotion decoding impairment is proposed as a possible integration of data coming from these different approaches.

Keywords: Facial recognition, emotion Rrecognition, brain science

Introduction

Asperger Syndrome (AS) is a neurodevelopmental disorder of social interaction within Autism Spectrum Disorders (ASD). In the last thirty years, the nosographic definition has increasingly proposed the autistic spectrum instead of distinct diagnostic profiles. The impulse from which this trend originated can be found in the acquisition of the dimensional model (Wing & Gould, 1979), forerunner of the DSM-5 proposal (Diagnostic and statistical manual of mental disorders [DSM]; 5th ed.; American Psychiatric Association [APA], 2013). Such proposal summarizes AS and other pervasive developmental disorders (PDD) (DSM-IV, 4th ed.; APA, 1994) in a unique autistic spectrum disorder diagnosis varying on a scale of gravity. In this perspective AS, already considered a form of High Functioning Autism (HFA), results as an entity of the same clinical continuum, of which autism would be the hard core (Prior et al., 1998). This change could refine the diagnostic criteria to better highlight the nuanced symptomatologic distinctions rather than uniforming them (Ghaziuddin, 2010).

Difficulties in social interaction and communication in individuals with normal intellectual capacity are described with a number of different diagnostic labels. It is unclear, however, whether they distinguish between separate syndromes, or simply describe the same morbid condition with different terminologies, according to the area of clinical competence. The term schizoid personality in childhood (Wolff & Chick, 1980), derived from psychotherapy, describes children with evident conduct disorders, better adaptation in adulthood, and slightly increased risk of schizophrenia. Nonverbal learning disabilities (NLD) (Rourke, 1989) are reported in neuropsychology and are described in neurology as developmental learning disabilities of the right hemisphere disorder (DLDRH) (Denckla, 1983; Weintraub & Mesulam, 1983). It has a deleterious impact on interactive and communicative styles and, consequently, on socialization skills.

The profound disturbances in emotional interpretation and expression, as well as in other basic interpersonal skills (Voeller, 1986), have subsequently a marked tendency to social withdrawal. It has been proposed that the similarities between the above described disorders may suggest a close relationship (Bejerot, 2007).

In the present chapter, only the terms ASD and AS will be used. These labels will be alternatively proposed to show common processes or, otherwise, to emphasize differences within the same spectrum.

Diagnostic criteria for Asperger's disorder according to DSM-IV (TR) (American Psychiatric Association 2000)

A. Qualitative impairment in social interaction, as manifested by at least two of the following:

1. marked impairment in the use of multiple non-verbal behaviours such as eye-to-eye gaze, facial expression, body postures, and gestures to regulate social interaction
2. failure to develop peer relationships appropriate to developmental level
3. a lack of spontaneous seeking to share enjoyment, interests, or achievements with other people (e.g. by a lack of showing, bringing, or pointing out objects of interest to other people)
4. lack of social or emotional reciprocity.

B. Restricted repetitive and stereotyped patterns of behaviour, interests, and activities, as manifested by at least one of the following:

1. encompassing preoccupation with one or more stereotyped and restricted patterns of interest that is abnormal either in intensity or focus
2. apparently inflexible adherence to specific, non-functional routines or rituals
3. stereotyped and repetitive motor mannerisms (e.g. hand or finger flapping or twisting, or complex whole-body movements)
4. persistent preoccupation with parts of objects.

C. The disturbance causes clinically significant impairment in social, occupational, or other important areas of functioning.

D. There is no clinically significant general delay in language (e.g. single words used by age two years, communicative phrases used by age three years).

E. There is no clinically significant delay in cognitive development or in the development of age-appropriate self-help skills, adaptive behaviour (other than in social interaction), and curiosity about the environment in childhood.

F. Criteria are not met for another specific Pervasive Developmental Disorder or Schizophrenia.

Figure 1. Diagnostic criteria for Asperger's disorder, DSM-IV (TR) (American Psychiatric Association, 2000).

As and Interactive Behaviors

AS diagnostics practice is based on behavioral data and clinical observations. The typical symptomatologic profile of AS individuals is characterized by a persistent qualitative impairment in mutual social and emotional interactions and by restricted, repetitive and stereotyped behaviors, interests and activities (DSM-IV-TR, 4th ed., text rev.; APA, 2000; see Fig. 1).

In addition, according to the typical perseverative behaviors displayed, these individuals exhibit signs of executive functions impairment, such as planning and organization, although their general cognitive abilities are preserved. Initial criteria included precocity in language learning ("he/she spoke even before walking"; Asperger, 1944 [as translated in Frith, 1991, pp. 37-92]), a particular fascination for letters and numbers, and sometimes the ability to decode words, although little or absent understanding (hyperlexia; Newman et al., 2007).

AS can establish attachment relationships to relatives, whereas approaches to peers and other people are inappropriate. Conversely to ASD, rather than retreat or remain detached, the child with AS can try to establish contacts with other children, hugging them or shouting, expressing amazement in response to their answers (Klin & Volkmar, 1995).

Regarding the social area, it is generally agreed that the alteration of mutual social and emotional interaction is the conditio sine qua non for both AS and ASD (Volkmar & Klin 2000). However, if compared to people with more severe forms of autism, individuals with AS are aware of the presence of others and are motivated to interact, frequently demonstrating a great interest in making friends and meeting people. Nevertheless, they show impairment in empathic resonance mechanisms, they have a limited usage of non-verbal language, such as eye contact, facial expressions, posture and gestures (McPartland & Klin, 2006); they have difficulties inferring feelings, intentions and nonverbal implicit communications of others (e.g., signs of boredom, haste to leave and need for privacy). Their speech can be often approximate or detailed, transmitting a sense of sketchy and inconsistent associations. In some cases, this may indicate a disorder of thought: the lack of consistency and reciprocity in speech is the result of a unilateral and self-centered conversational style. Thus, the latter assumes the form of an intense monologue about a particular topic, regardless of whether the other person is interested or not (Klin, McPartland, & Volkmar, 2005; Klin & Volkmar, 1995; Volkmar & Klin 2000; Wing, 1981). Verbose and tangential, their speech can also produce eccentric prosody in terms of volume, frequency or pace. Sometimes speech-breaks reflect the difficulty in formulating answers to questions and structuring the discourse (Woodbury-Smith & Volkmar, 2009).

Anyway, as scientific evidence seems to highlight, the central aspect of ASD concerns social competences, namely the individual's capacity to comprehend, coordinate and effectively use the personal available resources, depending on environmental, social and contextual characteristics. Thus, social competence appears as a superordinate and multidimensional construct which puts together different skills, while emotional abilities have a role of prominence and of close interconnection. As it has been observed, individuals with Typical Development (TD) begin to develop their skills to explore facial features and decode emotional expressions from the early days of their life (Schultz, 2005). In contrast, AS and ASD in general, lack eye contact and attention for the human face (Balconi & Carrera 2008; Grelotti, Gauthier, & Schultz, 2002; Marcus & Nelson 2001), and commonly display a dysfunction in affection-related behaviors, such as emotional reciprocity and emotional facial expressions decoding (Golarai, Grill-Spector, & Reiss, 2006).In short, the inability to recognize and embody emotions and feelings could generate a poor social cognition, which influences social skills in developing empathy and the possibility to successfully adapt to the social environment. In this context, facial expressions represent basic communicative signals of high interpersonal value with adaptive functions. In fact, emotional empathic behaviors include not only perception and action coupling, but also emotion sharing (Balconi & Canavesio, 2013a).

In the following paragraph, the salience of face stimuli in social life will be discussed and sustained by empirical evidence on control subjects. Moreover, some theoretical positions on emotion perception will be debated. These issues will be useful to better understand and ground social and emotional deficits in ASD, and specifically AS individuals, described in the last paragraphs.

Recognition of Facial Identity and Emotion

The human face represents one of the most important stimuli to convey and understand essential information for social interactions, and the capacity to perceive and respond to these cues is a turning point in social communication and behavior (Deeley et al., 2007). Faces are "probably the most visually complex, intrinsically meaningful visual stimuli with which we interact" (Elgar & Campbell, 2001), since they tell a lot about the identity of other individuals, as well as their emotional state, feelings and intentions (Balconi, Bortolotti, & Gonzaga, 2011; Balconi & Ferrari, 2012).

Considering all the visual perceptual skills in humans, face perception is considered to be the most developed one at all ages, starting from infancy, because faces are more prevalent and suggestive than other stimuli (Theeuwes & Van der Stigchel, 2006). After the first hours of birth newborns can recognize the mother's face (Bushnell, 2001) and are attracted by faces in general (Goren, Sarty, & Wu, 1975).

Studies on adults using modifications of the classic spatial cueing paradigm developed by Posner (1980) showed that faces can capture attention like exogenous events do, especially in case of threatening, or angry faces (Fox, Russo, Bowles, & Dutton, 2001), with a decrease in RTs for targets presented at the location that contains a face. In addition, a study by Ro, Russell and Lavie (2001) using a change blindness paradigm showed that participants prefer to look at faces rather than at objects, with a subsequent more rapid and accurate change detection. In fact, we need to prioritize faces rather than to look at them as generic objects, since they have a biological and phylogenetic relevance for humans safeguard (Balconi & Carrera, 2007). Moreover, Theeuwes and Van der Stigchel explored the inhibition of return (IOR) effect to show that faces can capture attention: IOR refers to a temporary suppression of orientation towards previously inspected location (Posner & Cohen, 1984). In this case, the authors observed the presence of delayed saccadic responses to a location that previously contained a face, arguing the presence of IOR for faces.

It has been underlined that faces represent a special, salient and meaningful stimulus for human interactions, so that they can influence and direct our attention. Much information is available from faces and many theoretical models have been proposed to account for the decoding process of these cues. Cognitive and neuropsychological models suggest different stages of facial processing, from perception to semantic identification, of which one of the best-known was developed by Bruce and Young (1998; see Fig. 2).

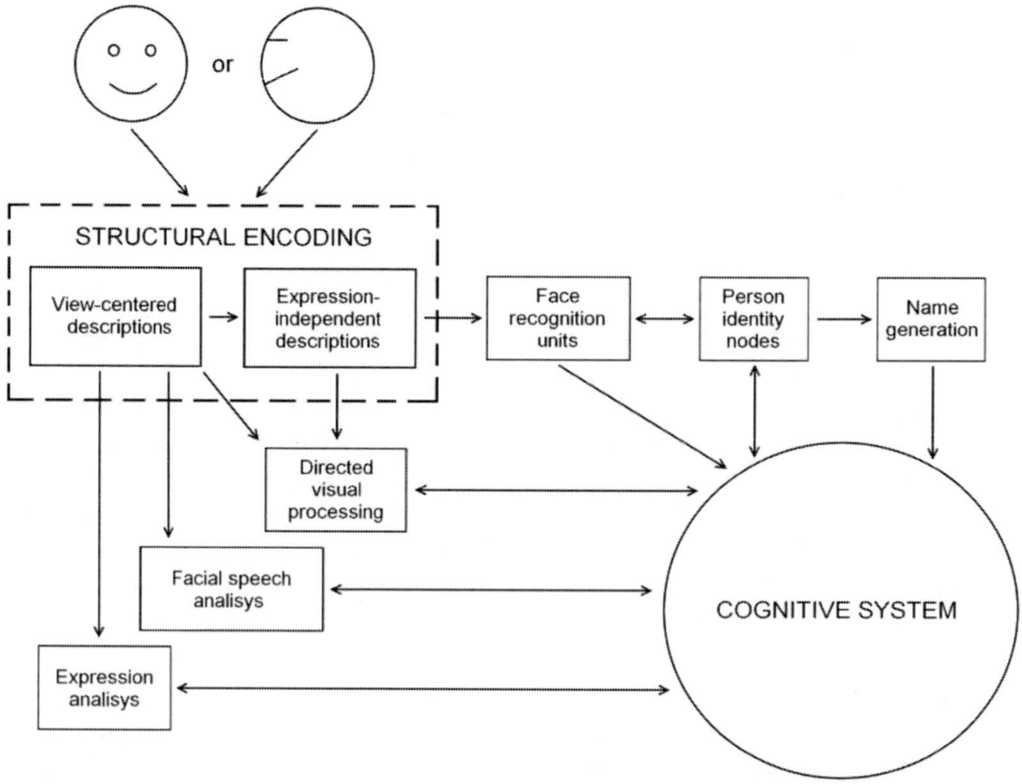

Figure 2. Bruce and Young model of face recognition (Bruce & Young, 1998).

This model has been expressed in terms of processing pathways and modules for the recognition of different kinds of information coming from a face. These cues are processed as "codes", with a sequential access to seven different codes: the pictorial, structural, visually derived semantics, identity-specific semantic, name, expression and facial speech ones (Balconi & Pozzoli, 2005, 2003). The pictorial code provides information about lighting, grain, pose and facial expression, shaping a 2D image of the face. The structural code, on the other hand, captures the aspects of the configuration of a face that distinguishes it from other faces: it corresponds to a 3D (view invariant) representation of the face. It is a more abstract visual representation that can mediate recognition (Balconi, 2008). This representation, in fact, is compared to pre-stored faces, with the selection and activation of the corresponding person identity node. Therefore, the model postulates that processing of familiar faces, because of the semantic hint, should be more automatic and rapid than that of unfamiliar ones, accompanied by more effort and longer reaction times. In this perspective it can be noted a dissociation between specific mechanisms that are responsible for the early structural encoding, and then higher-level mechanisms related to the integration of these representations within a semantic context. Hence, the model assumes functional independence between expression and identity processing and postulates that facial expressions are irrelevant for face recognition. However, some studies have challenged this assumption (Endo, Endo, Kirita, & Maruyama, 1992).

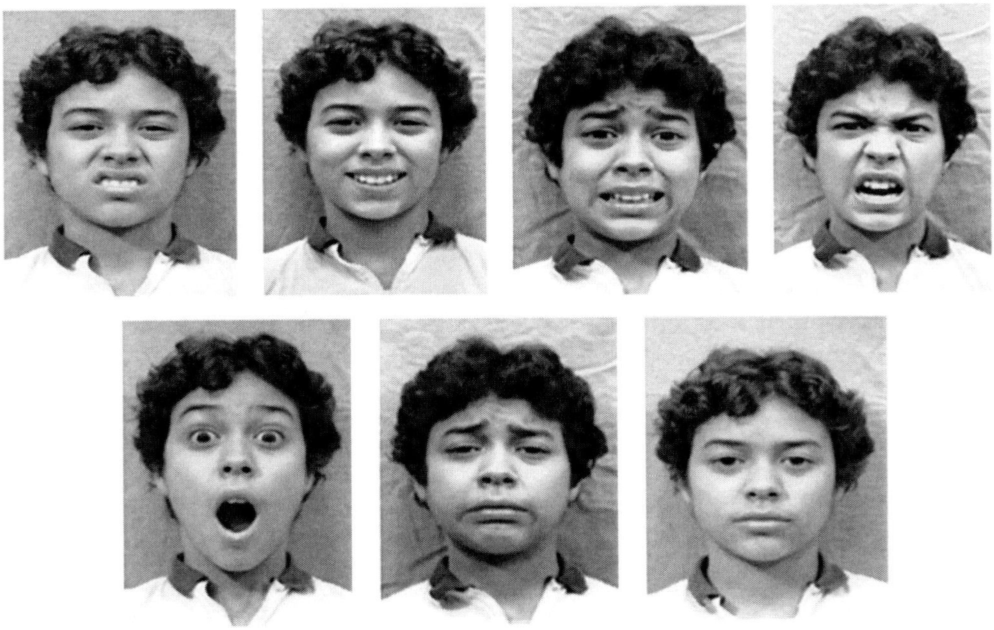

Figure 3. Examples of basic emotions (from left to right: disgust, happiness, fear, anger, surprise, sadness) and neutral expression.

Other authors tried to explain how faces are processed and encoded in the brain with the concept of Facial Prototypes. Solso and McCarthy (1981) proposed the idea of prototype formation to suggest that faces are encoded according to the statistics of their features, and then compared to the average of all the seen faces. The prototype stored in memory is "norm-based" and offers a flexible way to process faces by merely verifying differences from it, which is easier than separately encoding many and overlapping features of every single face (Or & Wilson, 2013). This allows taking advantage of the similarity between face exemplars, and, at the same time, to discriminate among subtle differences.

Besides the recognition of identity, people are very interested and skilled at understanding each other's facial expressions. Some research has shown that this is an early ability and that even neonates can respond to different facial expressions (Field, Woodson, Greenberg, & Cohen, 1982). One of the most controversial issues about facial expression recognition concerns the way emotions are recognized, and in particular whether they are perceived as qualitatively discrete categories or as varying along continuous dimensions (Hamann, 2012). Theories accounting for the first approach come from the evolutionary tradition, and one of the best known is supported by Paul Ekman (1992); such theories propose that we express and perceive a limited number of distinct emotion types, each with specific properties: happiness, sadness, anger, fear, disgust and surprise (See Fig. 3). Within this framework, basic emotions are considered to be universal, biologically determined, and to have specific physiological and neural profiles that distinguish them from one another.

On the other hand, the second theoretical position, represented by dimensional theories, conceptualizes emotions as the product of combinations of fundamental dimensions, such as emotional arousal (intensity of emotion) and valence (degree of pleasantness). One particular dimensional approach, termed the Circumflex Model of Affect (Russell, 1980), suggests that all affective states can be understood as a linear combination of two-dimensional and orthogonal bipolar dimensions, one related to valence (a pleasure-displeasure continuum) and the other to arousal, or alertness. Fear, for example, is conceptualized as the combination of negative valence and heightened arousal.

These dimensions are accompanied by both specific neurophysiological systems and cognitive interpretations of the emotional experience: the two underlying neurophysiological systems subserve all affective states, and upon this substrate various cognitive processes emerge to identify the neurophysiological changes in the valence and arousal systems. Interestingly, these processes allow interpreting the neurophysiological changes in relation to the eliciting stimuli, memories of prior experiences, behavioral responses and semantic knowledge (Russell, 2003). In this context, emotions could be seen as the product of a complex interaction between cognitions, likely occurring in neocortical structures, and neurophysiological changes related to the valence and arousal systems, which are presumably largely subserved by subcortical structures (Young et al.,1997).

Despite research's attempts to determine which of these theories better accounts for emotion expression and decoding, there remains a lack of consensus. Both theories relies on supportive psychophysiological data, which in one case show discriminable patterns of psychophysiological responses (Stephens, Christie, & Friedman, 2010), and in the other one account for consistent psychophysiological correlates of emotional arousal and valence dimensions (e.g., skin conductance response and facial muscle activity; Critchley, 2009).

Emotion Recognition in ASD and AS: Experimental Paradigms

With regard to children with autism, emotional recognition has been investigated by means of three main paradigms: sorting tasks, matching tasks and cross-modal identification. In sorting tasks, subjects are required to classify some pictures according to facial expression as well as to other criteria such as sex, age and type of hat. In matching tasks subjects are asked to match different pictures portraying emotional faces or non-emotional content. Finally, cross-modal paradigms require subjects to pair a specific facial expression with congruent cues from multiple communicative channels, for example voice, gesture or context (Balconi & Carrera, 2011).

It has been shown that, when submitted to a sorting task paradigm, ASD children choose non-emotional classification parameters like age, gender or type of hat to categorize presented faces (Davies, Bishop, Manstead, & Tantam, 1994). Moreover, they tend to ignore emotional expressions, even if explicitly required. In the matching task paradigm ASD individuals perform worse in conditions involving emotional faces pairing if compared, for example, to the identity condition (Celani, Battacchi, & Arcidiacono, 1999), while the opposite pattern is usually observed in non-autistic subjects. Finally, within cross-modal paradigm, it has been illustrated that individuals with ASD are less accurate than control individuals at matching an emotional voice to simultaneously presented dynamic emotional faces (Loveland, Tunali-Kotoski, Chen, Brelsford et al., 1995; Loveland, Tunali-Kotoski, Chen, Ortegon et al., 1997).

Other considerations about facial recognition in ASD children concern the way faces are explored as perceptual stimuli. It has been suggested that, unlike normally developing children, ASD subjects process faces in an analytical way, similar to the way they process objects, that is paying attention to every singular feature and relying more on local than global facial features of faces. In fact, it has been pointed out that autistics have an overall intact performance in face decoding when faces are presented inverted, with an equal number of correct answers for upright and upside down faces, while control children make significantly more errors when faces are presented inverted. The presentation of inverted faces, in fact, forces normal children to switch from the usual global processing of faces to a more analytical one (Deruelle, Rondan, Gepner, & Tardif, 2004). The lack of this effect in ASD children, well-known as the face-inversion effect, is considered a sign of a local, rather than a configural processing of faces (Carey & Diamond, 1994).

A diminished inversion-effect was also found in AS individuals: in a recent work Doi and colleagues (2013) explored the ability of adults with Asperger's Syndrome to process and recognize emotional categories of facial expressions and emotional prosodies according to their emotional intensity. They performed a recognition task in which photographs representing facial expressions with graded emotional intensities were presented upright or upside down to adults with and without AS. Results showed the presence of the classical inversion effect in both AS and control groups, for every emotional category. However, the magnitude of the inversion effect was diminished for angry and sad expressions in the Asperger group, who also outperformed in inverted sad expression recognition. This indicates a superior ability in people with AS, and ASD in general, to detect local facial information in recognizing facial expressions. Interestingly, the recognition abilities of facial expression were strongly influenced by the intensity of the emotional expressions: AS exhibited significantly poorer recognition abilities if compared to the control group for the stimuli with intermediate emotional intensities (60-80%), with delayed response speed, while the overall pattern of findings indicates that AS recognition capabilities are comparable with that of typically-developed controls for higher intensity emotional facial expressions.

The weakened inversion effect in ASD has been explained within the Weak Central Coherence Theory (Frith, 1989b), which supports the idea of a general perceptive deficit, focalizing the attention on their difficulties in creating coherent representations of their context (Frith, 2003). Empirical evidence shows that normal children's processing takes advantage from the occurrence of meaningful and patterned information, whereas ASD people seem to show a reduction or absence of this benefit, from meaning or central coherence (Happé & Frith, 1996). In addition, besides perceptive processing, this effect would also influence language and memory functions: Frith (1989a) reviewed and reinterpreted early works on ASD skills and found that in memory recall tasks normal children recall meaningful sentences better than random word strings, whereas ASD children don't show this advantage, and are almost equally good with both linguistic stimuli (Hermelin & O'Connor, 1967; Tager-Flusberg, 1991). As far as meaning comprehension, normal subjects can extract the concept of a passage or story while forgetting the surface form (Bartlett, 1932); on the contrary, ASD people may precisely retain the words used but fail to deduce meaning.

The idea that people with autism make relatively less use of global information and pay preferential attention to parts rather than wholes, can account for both deficit and advantages in autism: Shah and Frith (1993) investigated the well-known block design skill in ASD children and found that this superior performance is largely due to an advantage in segmenting the original design, as if they would see the configuration in terms of its constituent parts. Interestingly, the presentation of pre-segmented patterns to normal controls significantly improved their performance, eliminating inter-groups differences in the task. In the same way, subjects with autism perform better than controls in visual illusions tasks, since controls are captured by figure context (Happé, 1996a).

Since it seems that weak central coherence entails benefits as well as disadvantages, it has been proposed that this aspect of autism could be genetically transmitted and that it could characterize an extended phenotype of autism, marking out some of the non-autistic relatives. Findings of superior block design and less coherent narrative in ASD relatives support this hypothesis (Landa, Folstein, & Isaacs, 1991; Smalley & Asarnow, 1990). Considering the socio-emotional field, this tendency to focalize on details and the difficulty to create a global representation of different components could impede the extraction of a global meaning in decoding facial emotional expressions (Frith, 2003).

Automatic System Contribution in Facial Expression Recognition

The same experimental paradigms described so far have been applied in emotions studies in ASD together with autonomic system activity recordings. In fact, besides behavioral measures, this method could be very promising in that it allows for a more direct way to explore emotions and social reciprocity. When an individual perceives motivationally relevant stimuli, such as emotional faces, a variety of specific emotional processes emerge in peripheral nervous system. Skin Conductance Response (SCR) is thought to reflect the arousal associated with the presentation of salient, socially-relevant and motivationally significant stimuli (Lang, Bradley, & Cuthbert, 1990), such as emotional faces or scenes.

Mathersul, McDonald and Rushby (2013a) applied this technique in emotional tasks involving ASD individuals and found systematic anomalies in peripheral indexes. Healthy controls displayed the typical pattern of higher SCRs to affective versus neutral stimuli and showed the expected differentiation for affective startle, with the pleasant stimuli eliciting a greater evoked cardiac acceleration response (ECA) than unpleasant stimuli. In fact, in control subjects startle reflexes are increased when the participant is exposed to unpleasant stimuli and weakened when exposed to pleasant stimuli (Mathersul et al., 2013a).

Adults with ASD showed atypical autonomic responses to extreme social affective patterns and specifically, rather than differentiating stimuli according to their valence, they displayed an overall dampening in SCRs in both affective conditions, but not in response to neutral images. The authors have interpreted this effect as implying a failure to orient to socially relevant stimuli and as a greater attribution of significance to neutral versus affective images. Moreover, besides the activation responses to emotional stimulation, the authors were also interested in exploring the presence of a direct relationship between baseline arousal levels (Skin Conductance Level, SCL) and the behavioral profiles of adults with ASD (Mathersul, McDonald, & Rushby, 2013b). Findings showed the presence of different subgroups within the ASD group according to differences in resting SCL. Such differences were accompanied by specific behavioral profiles. Specifically, the ASD group with significantly lower resting SCL also showed poorer recognition and judgment capabilities of basic emotions, while the ASD group with typical resting SCL did not differ from controls.

Thus, it has been shown that results coming from studies adopting implicit measures of social engagement are particularly useful in that they are thought to influence subsequent behavioral responses in experimental settings, as well as in everyday life.

Attentional Mechanisms and Emotional Salience of Faces

As already discussed, ASD children report a reduction in social attention and an increase in visual attention to nonsocial stimuli. Then, emotional and motivational significance of facial expressions may also result in changes of motivated attention (Balconi & Pozzoli, 2009).

Eye movements reveal important information about one person's interests and subsequently about the salience of a presented stimulus. Then, eye tracking could provide another implicit measure of ASD's emotional orienting and engagement. In a recent study Sasson and Touchstone (2014) performed a visual paired preference task consisting of twenty paired faces and object images. Objects were interestingly manipulated by the authors and were both related to common stuff (furniture, clothing, tools, musical instruments and plants) and also to the most frequently occurring topics of circumscribed interest in ASD (trains, vehicles, airplanes, clocks and blocks). Findings showed that preschoolers with ASD performed similarly to control subjects if the face was presented together with common objects. This finding is particularly relevant in that it shows that they did not exhibit an absolute deficit in social attention or actively avoid attending to faces. On the contrary, ASD performed more poorly than control subjects if presented with objects related to circumscribed interests, suggesting that social attention in ASD preschoolers could be modulated by the salience of competing non-social stimuli. This distinction has important implications because it accounts for a relative unbalance between social and nonsocial attention from a very early age: such unbalance may indicate a link between social and repetitive behavior domains of ASD.

Results showing poorer recognition performance in emotional facial expressions in ASD have also been replicated for individuals with High-Functioning Autism (HFA) and AS (Humphreys, Minshew, Leonard, & Behrmann, 2007; Kätsyri, Saalasti, Tiippana, Von Wendt, & Sams, 2008; Law, Montagne, Perrett, Gill, & Gallagher, 2010); Hanley, McPhillips, Mulhern, and Riby (2013) explored attention allocation to faces in adolescents with Asperger Syndrome using the eye-tracker and a range of static faces viewed either in isolation or in the context of a social scene. Findings showed that faces were viewed typically by the individuals with Asperger's Syndrome when presented in isolation, but attention to the eyes was significantly diminished in comparison to control participants when faces were viewed as part of social scenes. In this case, in fact, there was additional information competing for attention. The author proposed two possible explanations for this result, the first accounting for social perception, and the second for social cognition explanation. According to a social-perceptual explanation, participants with AS may exhibit reduced attention to the eyes because their vision may be captured by other visual information. Alternatively, a social cognitive account attributes the need, for control subjects, to look at the eyes to understand the social interaction, while the same need could not be that urgent in AS. This study demonstrated that participants with AS can exhibit either typical or atypical attentional patterns to the eye region of faces depending on the nature of stimuli, and suggests that a possible cause of discrepancy in research findings could be attributable to the use of different stimuli. It is thought that these behaviors are due to a lack of motivational commitment in people with ASD, which would result in a reduced attention to social stimuli like faces, but also to voice and hands gestures (Dawson, Webb, & McPartland, 2005; Grossman, Klin, Carter, & Volkmar, 2000; Mathersul et al., 2013a; Oberman, Winkielman, & Ramachandran, 2009).

Marotta and colleagues (2013) explored more automatic and implicit indices of attention to social information in people with and without Asperger's Syndrome, and in particular the IOR effect (See Par. 2) for eye-gaze direction and peripheral cues, either congruent or incongruent with target presentation. The authors described the eye-gaze and the peripheral cues as social and non-social signals, respectively. Impairment in IOR effects for gaze cues was observed in the Asperger group, who responded faster to targets presented in locations previously cued by eye-gaze direction, whereas typically developing participants showed the expected effect. On the other hand, peripheral cues elicited comparable levels of IOR between individuals with autism and the matched comparison group. The authors explained these findings as consistent with the impairment in social attention and suggest the eye gaze as a special stimulus to study social attention.

It has to be noted that it is still not clear whether these deficits are directly responsible for the impairment observed in emotional behavior, or if difficulties in decoding emotions lead to a lack of interest for the human face.

Brain Correlates and Event-Related Potentials (ERP) Studies in Facial Expression Recognition

The perception of a highly salient stimulus is also been accompanied by central system indicators of emotional processing. Deeley and colleagues (2007) investigated the effect of emotion intensity on recognition processing within an implicit event-related fMRI . This technique is particularly useful in that it allows measuring and precisely localizing the brain activity associated with a cerebral function, in the form of changes in blood oxygenation. In this case, AS and healthy controls were required to press a button to decide upon the sex of each fearful, disgusted, happy and sad face. Results revealed fusiform (Fusiform Gyrus, FG; Fusiform Face Area, FFA) and extrastriate activations in both AS and control participants, with positive trends of activation to increasing emotional intensity of faces, and in particular of fear and happiness. Further, if compared to controls, AS showed reduced activation in these areas. Despite some differences between conditions, this hyporesponsiveness persisted across emotion types and intensities. As a possible explanation of these findings the authors suggested that this pattern could reflect a failure of feedback modulation from limbic structures in people with AS. This suggestion is consistent with those theories that attribute emotional and social deficits to structural and functional abnormalities of specific brain areas (Baron-Cohen et al., 2000; Howard et al., 2000). In fact, during the presentation of highly emotional facial expressions, healthy controls recruit brain areas involved in face processing networks, such as fusiform and limbic regions (Surguladze et al., 2003).

Specifically, the visual cortex activation would be sustained by feedback influences from the amygdala (Morris et al., 1998). The presence of such activation could emerge in an increasing detection, prioritization, and memorization of meaningful social cues (Vuilleumier,

Richardson, Armony, Driver, & Dolan, 2004). Neuroimaging literature on facial emotion perception and recognition in ASD reports anomalies, in terms of reduced limbic and FG activation, as compared to healthy controls (Critchley et al., 2000).

Baron-Cohen and colleagues (2000) proposed the Amygdala Theory of Autism, suggesting that abnormalities in this brain region could explain ASD social and emotional impairment. In fact, within an fMRI study, they found significantly lower activation in the amygdala region during a mentalizing task in adults with HFA and AS, if compared to controls (Baron-Cohen et al., 1999). The experiment consisted in the presentation of two visual tasks involving the comprehension of socially relevant information from facial stimuli. Participants were asked to decide for each stimulus which of two simultaneously presented words best described the gender or the mental state of the subject, alternatively. Results related to the mentalizing task showed a less extensively activation of the frontal region in ASD group, which also didn't activate the amygdala at all. Meanwhile, they exhibited significantly greater activation in the bilateral Superior Temporal Gyrus (STG). This finding is relevant in that it suggests the presence of compensation strategies to amygdala abnormalities: in fact it seems that AS recur to linguistic components and structures specialized for verbally label these complex visual stimuli.

Baron-Cohen (2002) suggested that, on a functional level, the way AS individuals process faces can be termed "systemizing", in that they tend to focus more on details and rules in order to rationally infer what other individuals are feeling, rather than automatically "empathizing" with their emotional state (Baron-Cohen et al., 1999; Baron-Cohen, 2002). From an ontogenetic perspective, it has been proposed that the dysfunction in the amygdala-fusiform system could occur during a critical period of early development (Schultz, 2005). Besides these cerebral regions, neuroimaging research has also pointed out the presence of hypoactivation in the Medial Prefrontal Cortex (MPFC) (Castelli, Frith, Happé, & Frith, 2002; Happé et al., 1996), which is involved in tasks implying mentalization, meta-cognition and empathy (Frith & Frith, 2003).

ASD's recourse to a more verbal thinking during face recognition tasks has also been found in EEG studies. Yang, Savostyanov, Tsai, and Liou (2011) compared EEG reactions of AS and healthy participants within an emotion recognition task; event-related spectral perturbation (ERSP) was applied to characterize the oscillatory activity in both groups. EEG rhythms are the result of synchronized activity within neuronal assemblies and the occurrence of changes in EEG power is thought to reflect changes in neuronal synchrony. Then, time-frequency analyses provide useful information about the neurophysiological modifications induced by an experimental task. Results showed two component of Theta power increase (4-8 Hz) following the face presentation in healthy subjects. This effect was weaker in AS participants for both the early and late reactions. The synchronization in this frequency range could be interpreted as an indicator of face emotion recognition. Interestingly, emotion-related theta synchronization is connected with the activity of the amygdala (Horel, Keating, & Misantone, 1975). Thus, the group differences in this band activity could reflect an impairment in the cortico-subcortical network involved in automatic emotion recognition in AS, as previously discussed. Moreover, control participants exhibited a desynchronization of Alpha and Beta rhythms over the posterior region, which has been traditionally interpreted as an indicator of directed attention to stimuli (Balconi & Pozzoli, 2009; Tranel & Hyman, 1990). In this case AS showed a significantly stronger desynchronization in the Alpha and Beta 2 range. Several empirical data showed that beta desynchronization is stronger in tasks requiring verbal thinking. Accordingly, the strengthened Beta 2 activity in AS could be interpreted as an indicator of more intensive participation of voluntary attention and verbal thinking in the face recognition processing.

In this framework, EEG reactions of AS participants may suggest an impairment in elementary functions, represented by a weaker Theta synchronization, and the recourse to a more intensive use of voluntary functions, reflected by the increased Beta 2 desynchronization. In fact, according to an evolutionary interpretation of EEG rhythms, slow wave (Delta and Theta) oscillations relies on phylogenetically ancient structures responsible for execution of automatic brain functions, such as the automatic recognition of emotions, whereas higher frequency rhythms (Alpha and Beta) are generated in later-forming structures during the execution of higher, voluntary-controlled mental functions (Aggleton, 1992).

Evidence of impaired processing of facial stimuli in ASD has also emerged within ERP paradigms: event-related potentials (ERPs) are small voltage shifts generated in specific brain structures in response to events or mental operations. Thanks to the high temporal resolution, ERPs can be very useful to trace the time course of neural information processes involved in particular mental operations. Within ASD literature, the absence of the typical inversion effect emerged on either N170 latency or amplitude (Grice et al., 2001; McPartland, Dawson, Webb, Panagiotides, & Carver, 2004) in comparison to typically-developing controls. N170 is a negative ERP component occurring at around 140-200 ms that is largest in response to human faces relative to objects (Itier & Taylor, 2002). The effect is particularly evident over posterior-temporal areas. Within an ERP study, O'Connor, Hamm, and Kirk (2007) asked AS and control participants to discriminate between neutral and sad expressions. Findings showed that, although AS could correctly recognize facial expressions as accurately as controls, they exhibited delayed N170 latencies to these stimuli. Also, this delay did not occur in response to objects. Control participants, on the other side, showed earlier N170 effect to faces if compared to object-related responses. Considering the N170 as an index of configural face processing (Balconi & Pozzoli, 2005; Eimer, 2000), the authors suggested that the delay to faces in AS adults may reflect slower processing of facial information or, alternatively, it may underline the lower experience at processing face and facial configuration in this population (Pelphrey et al., 2002).

Considering another level of analysis, Balconi, Amenta, and Ferrari (2012) investigated emotional competencies of control, autistic and Asperger children exploring their linguistic and conceptual skills during the presentation of emotional faces, pictures and videos (See Fig. 4 a,b). Subjects were required to identify the emotion and to explain possible causes of the emotional state; then, a semantic analysis was performed focusing on conceptualization and labelling. Starting from conceptualization, ASD children described the emotional cues focusing more prominently on inanimate objects, and less on characters or interactive situations while, as expected, the opposite pattern was observed for control children. The AS group presented a pattern more similar to that of control group, even if an increased interest for objects was also observed.

As far as what concerns labelling, instead, results showed that while control participants were capable of labeling correctly all emotional categories with an appropriate and relevant verbal production, responses within the ASD group were different: Asperger participants showed preserved abilities to correctly label all emotional dimensions with the exception of surprise, whereas autistic participants showed clear impairments in decoding disgust, surprise and, in part, sadness. However, verbal production of both autistic and Asperger individuals was quite appropriate and relevant for all the emotional correlates, with the exception of surprise.

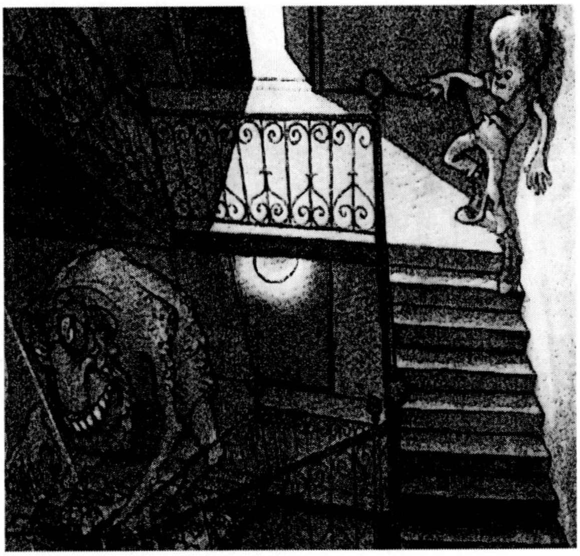

a

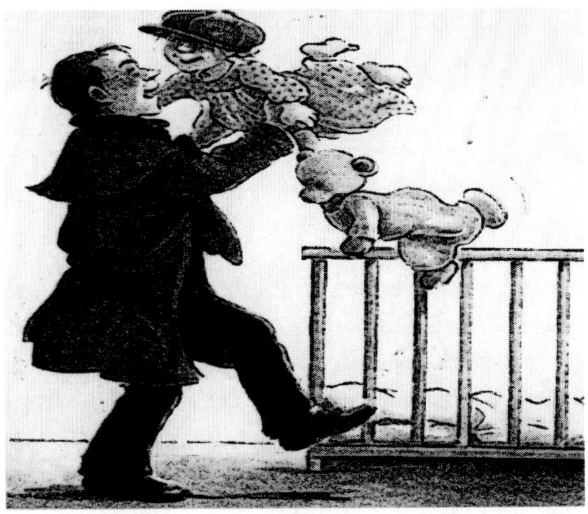

b

Figure 4. Examples of emotional scripts of a) fear and b) happiness used in empirical research (Balconi & Carrera 2007, mod.).

The inability to correctly recognize surprise might be linked both to different face processing strategies and also to a mentalizing deficit; since it has been shown that ASD subjects tend to focus mainly on the lower part of the face (Klin, Jones, Schultz, Volkmar, & Cohen, 2002), the first hypothesis relies on the fact that this pattern of analysis might be difficult for these subjects in that the analysis of both mouth and eye elements is necessary. The mentalization hypothesis, instead, relies on that empirical evidence which showed that ASD, and in particular HFA and AS individuals, maintain preserved abilities in recognizing at least basic emotions like happiness or sadness (Balconi et al., 2012; Loveland et al., 1997). This preservation has been explained with the distinction between first-order and second-order processes: specifically, emotions like happiness or sadness can be easily interpreted recurring to simple first-order representational process mostly based on contextual information, while complex emotions like surprise need the intervention of second-order meta-representation processes, which are impaired in ASD. According to this interpretation, surprise could be considered a belief-based emotion instead of a reality-based emotion (Baron-Cohen, Spitz, & Cross, 1993). In fact, the difficulty to recognize surprise was the real discriminant between the clinical and the control group: this suggests a development of emotional competencies proceeding from the recognition of basic emotions (e.g., happiness and anger) to the acquisition of more complex ones (e.g., surprise).

As can be noted, like for studies with ASD, results on emotions perception in AS have reported controversial findings, depending on the type of stimuli, paradigm and level of analysis. It should be underlined that, in some circumstances, the performance of control and AS individuals is comparable, thus accounting for the preservation of some emotional skills. In general, research indicates that high-functioning autistic and AS individuals have preserved abilities to recognize basic emotions like happiness or sadness (Balconi et al., 2012), according to a hierarchical conception of acquisition of emotional capabilities. Moreover, it seems that AS individuals process faces focusing on details and rules, rather than empathizing with their emotional state (Baron-Cohen et al., 1999). In this context, recent research claims for underestimated social and emotional capabilities in autistic children.

For example, Jemel, Mottron, and Dawson (2006), within an exhaustive review of behavioral, ERP and functional imaging studies, maintain that for several aspects face processing abilities of autistic individuals did not differ from their typical developed skills.

Theory of Mind and Social Skill Impairment

The ability to understand people's mental states and emotions and the capacity to assign mental states to others has been defined as theory of mind. The affective component of these capabilities has often been described as empathy (Baron-Cohen, 2002), and it is reported to be impaired in individuals with ASD (Baron-Cohen, 1995). Mentalizing abilities develop since the first years of life; the child gradually acquires the capacity to empathize and perceive others' mental and affective states through different stages. Referential gaze, joint attention, declarative pointing and symbolic game are considered early precursors of more complex social and emotional competencies, including the ability to decode, understand and predict intentions, actions and motivations. These opportunities to access shared emotional meanings can improve the relational world (Baron-Cohen, 1995, 2002). A specific deficit at this level could affect verbal and nonverbal communication and produce difficulties in the establishing of mutual social interactions.

Baron-Cohen (1995) summarized the perspective of Theory of Mind (ToM) with the term "mind blindness." Within this theory, ASD are considered to live in a world where they can't understand that other people experience different mental states (e.g., believes, desires) and that their behaviors are strictly related to these states (Baron-Cohen, 1989a, 1995; Baron-Cohen, Leslie, & Frith, 1985; Leslie, 1991; Leslie & Keeble, 1987; Leslie & Roth, 1993). This would limit their social reciprocity, leaving the individual in the mind blindness state.

Empirical evidence supports this theoretical perspective: in particular, ToM has been tested employing false-belief paradigms: in these tasks children are required to make predictions on possible outcomes related to specific situations, which could be inferred only by engaging in first or second-order meta-representational reasoning (Baron-Cohen et al., 1985). In these tasks, autistic children perform worse than typically-developing children, and it has been suggested that they may have a deficient or delayed ToM (Baron-Cohen et al., 1985). ASD individuals, in fact, exhibit an impairment in the comprehension of others' affective experience when the evaluation requires the representation of their beliefs and causal factors, which constitute the most explanatory elements of emotional experience (Want & Harris, 2001).

Further evidence supporting ToM comes, for example, from the Faux Pas Test (Baron-Cohen et al., 1999). This paradigm has proven that, despite the capability to solve first and second order false-belief tasks, ASD show impairment in the comprehension of the emotional and psychological impact related to a faux pas. In the same way, moral reasoning tasks revealed that ASD have difficulties in judging the intentionality of an action, although being able to detect incorrectness or a wrong scene. In fact, they can't consider the gaffe as unintentional and tend to blame the protagonist as if he or she would have behaved intentionally (Zalla & Leboyer, 2011; Zalla, Sav, Stopin, Ahade, & Leboyer, 2009), especially in the case of immoral actions ("Knobe effect"; Knobe, 2003). In this case, they attribute greater importance to normative transgressions rather than to the person's intentions (Zalla et al., 2009). Even if it is widely accepted and appreciated, ToM explanation has been submitted to some criticism. In a recent study Kamio, Wolf, and Fein (2006) performed an affective priming task to investigate the autonomic response to emotional faces and non-emotional objects in high-functioning individuals with autism. Participants were also required to label emotional expressions. Findings showed that they were able to discriminate emotional faces, even if they didn't exhibit the affective priming effect. Authors suggested that this atypical response is due to a failure in evaluating the significance of emotional faces and not a failure in understanding other people mental states, as supposed by the ToM approach. In fact Kamio's study revealed that also automatic processing of simple emotions was atypical, even if they had no difficulties in categorize them. Actually, it seems that their level of cognitive ability allows them to use compensatory strategies.

Empathy and the Mirror Neuron System

A more recent theory tried to explain social and emotional difficulties in individuals with ASD with the disruption of more automatic and spontaneous processes: this theory argues that one of the causes of social impairment in autism could lie on an early dysfunction of the "mirror neuron system" and that this is the primary cause of the whole spectrum of social disabilities characterizing autism, including facial expressions decoding (Dapretto et al., 2006; Ramachandran & Oberman, 2006). Emotion processing and emotional face detection are central mechanisms that allow subjects to adequately respond to the perceived emotion, by simulating the affective state of others and mirroring the observed emotional behavior (Balconi & Bortolotti, 2013a). The mirror neuron system, in fact, seems to represent the neural mechanism underlying simulation processes that allow the embodiment of social understanding and empathetic response (Gallese, 2005; Keysers & Gazzola, 2006). This hypothesis found support on empirical findings showing autistic children's inability to succeed in automatic imitation tasks, and gave birth to the "broken-mirror" theory of autism (Dapretto et al., 2006; Ramachandran & Oberman, 2006). In normal development, the ability to mimic is fundamental to capture other people's emotions: when viewing emotional facial expressions, children spontaneously activate the same muscles and mimic each other's actions and emotional displays. This ability is called "automatic mirroring" and occurs quickly and without voluntary control (Lundquist & Dimberg, 1995). This is also thought to facilitate social interactions, interpersonal relationships, and emotions recognition (Balconi & Bortolotti, 2012; Lundquist & Dimberg, 1995). However, this spontaneous mimicry appears to be lacking in children with autism (Rogers, Hepburn, Stackhouse, & Wehner, 2003). Moreover, they show abnormal activation of brain areas related to the mirror neuron system, and specifically to intentional attention allocation and categorization processes (Hall, Szechtman, & Nahmias, 2003).

It has been shown, on the basis of anatomical (Hadjikani, Joseph, Snyder, & Tager-Flusberg, 2006) and neurophysiological (Dapretto et al., 2006; Nishitani, Avikainen, & Hari, 2004) evidence, that this system is highly activated during imitation tasks or tasks involving automatic-mimicry processes. Several studies have shown that ASD individuals, including AS and HFA, display delayed or absent spontaneous facial expressions of happiness and anger, whereas their voluntary facial expressions remain intact (Beall, Moody, McIntosh, Hepburn, & Reed, 2008; Hermans, Van Wingen, Bos, Putman, & Van Honk, 2009; McIntosh, Reichmann-Decker, Winkielman, & Wilbarger, 2006; Oberman et al., 2009).

More recent studies suggested that the mimic impairments reported in autism may only be affected for the automatic component of mimicry, since they fail to imitate non-goal-oriented actions and gestures. On the other hand, autistic children show normal performance during the imitation of goal-oriented actions, meaningful objects, or facial expressions (Rogers et al., 2003; Stone, Ousley, & Littleford, 1997). Rogers, Hepburn, Stackhouse, and Wehner (2003) suggested that mimicry in autism might involve two distinct processes: an affective mechanism which spontaneously and automatically modulates social interactions and a second intentional mechanism mediated by executive functions and meta-cognitive processes. Current evidence shows that autistic children have consistent impairment in automatic mimicry while preserving the ability to understand and imitate goal-directed actions (Hall et al., 2003). In this framework, it is possible to hypothesize that autistic children recur to the intentional imitation system to compensate the impairment of automatic processes. However, this hypothesis has been recently criticized by Hamilton (2008), who maintained that a theory of a global breakdown of the mirror neuron system is not able to explain the complexity of the data in autistic research. In fact, since the mirror neuron system is involved in a variety of tasks beyond automatic mimicry, we should expect impairment in other cognitive tasks such as imitation of goal-directed actions or understanding of actions' goals. Hamilton, instead, proposed that the neural pathway supporting goal representation might be spared in autism while the functioning of the direct path may be compromised, with a subsequent reduction in the child's ability to spontaneously imitate gestures or facial expressions (Oberman et al., 2009).

A Multi-Functional Impairment and Underconnectivity Model

We have pointed out that emotion decoding and understanding is a complex process, in that its acquisition involves social, cognitive and neural domains. Face-processing impairment in autism spectrum disorders has been described as a result of neurocognitive development, a perceptual deficit, as well as a consequence of reduced interest in social stimuli. Hence, the available literature and the empirical findings suggest that face decoding impairment can't be exclusively attributed to cognitive, social or neural factors. Instead, it may be more easily and extensively understood as the result of a complex integration between these factors, detected at different levels of analysis. Consequently, a failure of emotion comprehension process can't be exhaustively explained if not referring to multiple and qualitative different factors.

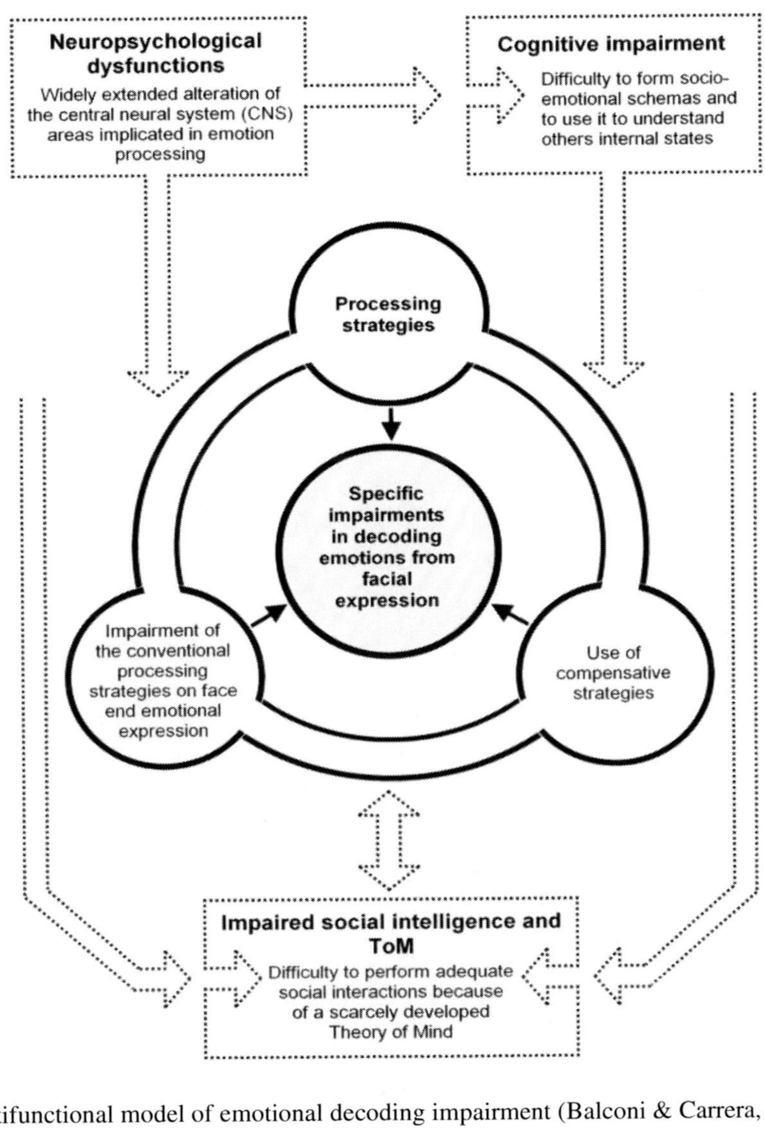

Figure 5. Multifunctional model of emotional decoding impairment (Balconi & Carrera, 2008, mod.).

In 2008 Balconi and Carrera proposed an integrate view that tried to incorporate evidence of emotional face comprehension impairment in ASD by means of a new conceptualization, in order to provide a comprehensive perspective on the phenomenon (see Fig. 5). This model illustrates the complex interactions of different factors that contribute to explain the deficits in recognizing and understanding emotions on the basis of facial expression cues. At the core of the model lies the specific impairment in decoding emotions from facial expressions, deriving from a deficiency in conventional processing strategies of face and emotional expressions and relying on both neuropsychological and cognitive dysfunctions. These functions interact with social intelligence and ToM.

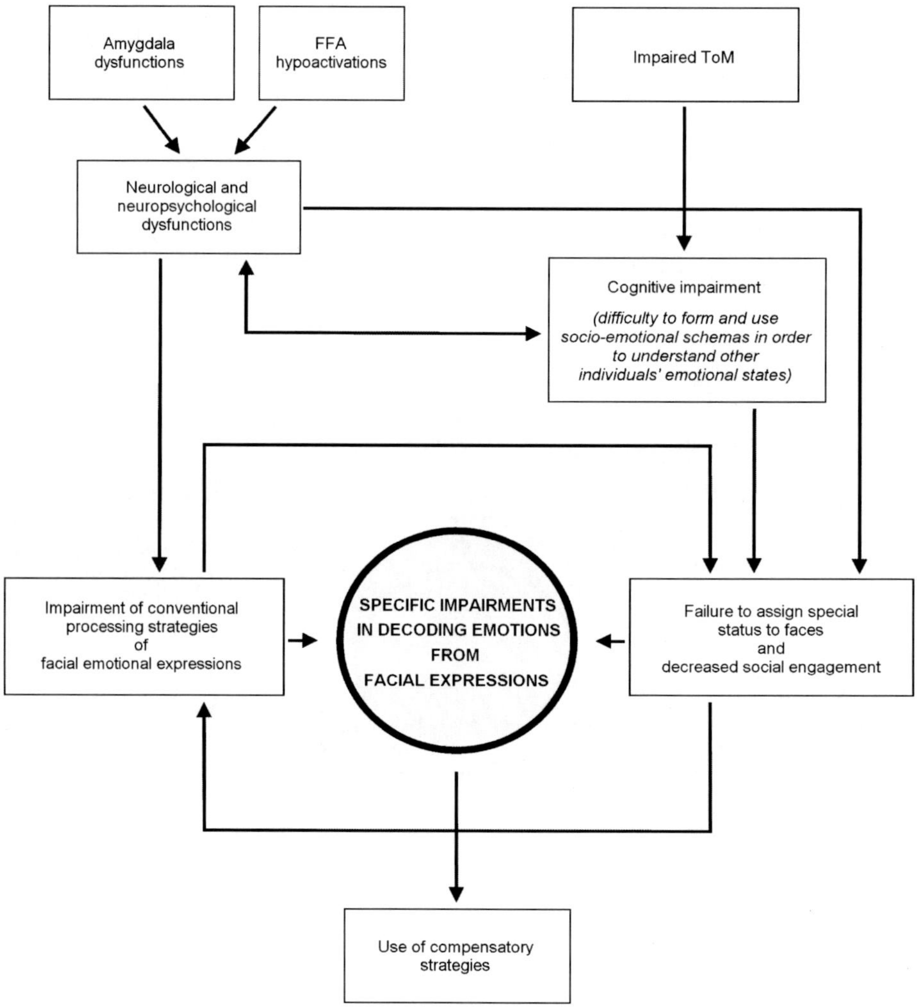

Figure 6. Multifunctional model of emotional decoding impairment modified to include specific patterns of neurological deficits. It suggests that specific impairments observed in emotional decoding in autism are the effect of the interaction between neural, social, and cognitive impairments (Amenta, Ferrari & Balconi, 2014).

The model has been recently modified and revised by Amenta, Ferrari, and Balconi (2014). The new version has been conceived within a more structured and interactive model, with stronger significance to neuropsychological evidence (see Fig. 6).

In fact, as previously discussed, the literature indicates that face processing is mediated by very early visual experience and perceptual skills (Grelotti et al., 2005; Schultz, 2005). It is therefore possible that earlier functional abnormalities involving perceptual systems and the amygdala could contribute to faces' lack of salience. This could be either the origin or the consequence of the social deficit shown in autism, according to a bidirectional pathway.

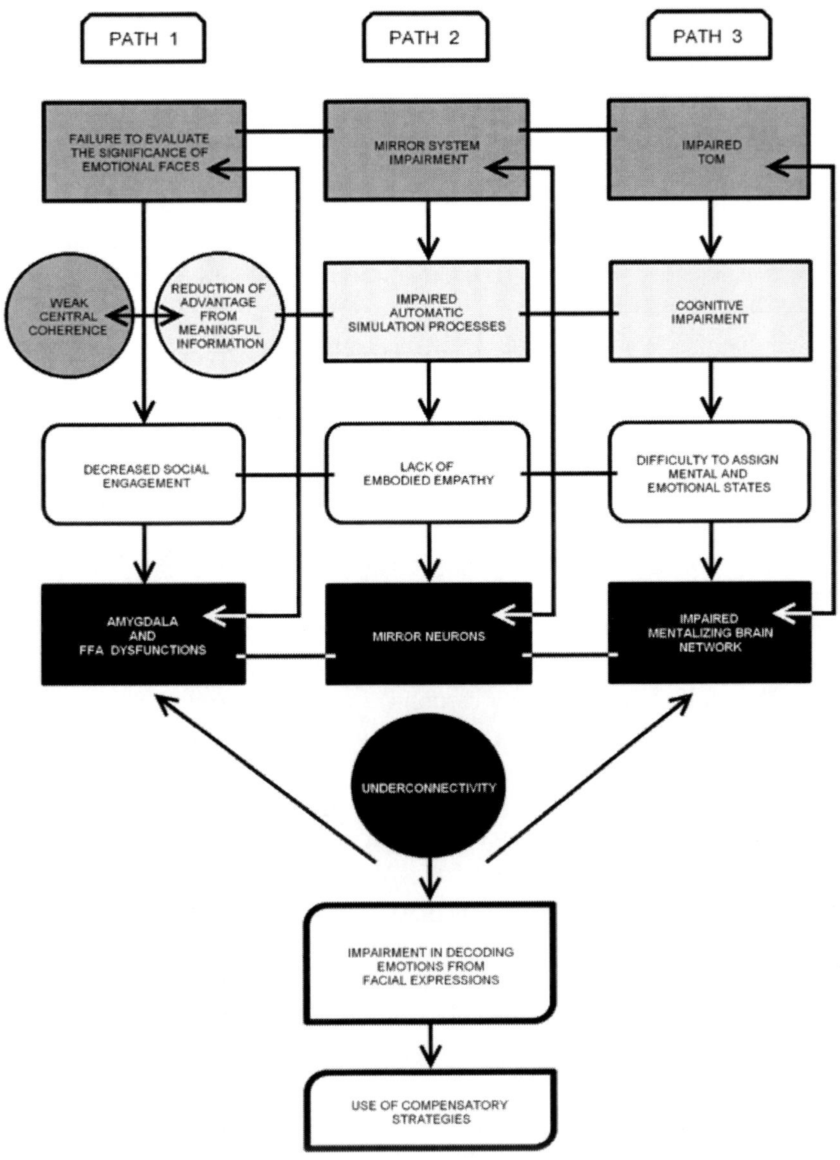

Figure 7. Multifunctional model of facial emotional decoding impairment revised here to distinguish between functions, competencies, symptoms and neural correlates (from top to bottom, respectively) and to suggest the involvement of three different pathways (1-3, from left to right) in facial emotion comprehension.

As far as what concerns cognitive impairment, in this case it has been attributed to impaired ToM, and it has been thought to reciprocally interact with functional abnormalities of the abovementioned brain areas. This model is particularly interesting in that it underlines, as a possible outcome of these impairments, the presence of compensatory strategies.

Here a renewed version of the model is proposed (see Fig. 7), emerging from a multi-functional approach.

Exploring the diagram from the top to the bottom it is possible to find a first distinction between functions, competencies, symptoms and neural correlates respectively, which constitutes a first element of novelty if compared to previous versions of the model. In addition, the contribution of these different levels is better specified in the light of the most recent empirical evidences. Moreover, a second distinction includes the presence three pathways (1-3), which are set from the left to the right. We discuss this second novel element in detail.

The first pathway concerns the evaluation of the emotional significance of faces. In fact, as already discussed, it has been proven that this function is impaired in ASD; according to the model, the impairment of this function would account for the reduced benefit from meaningful information coming from faces. Moreover, it could explain the preferential attention given to parts rather than wholes, and the subsequent reduced inversion effect, as already suggested by the Weak Central Coherence Theory (Happé & Frith, 1996). The development of these competencies serves as an interface for a proficient social involvement, which is also compromised in the case of ASD individuals. The proposed neural correlates for the first pathway lie in the amygdala and the FFA, which have been proven to allow for the detection and prioritization of meaningful social cues (Vuilleumier et al., 2004) and to be less activated in ASD (Critchley et al., 2000). The operation of these brain areas is strictly linked to the difficulties in evaluating the emotional significance from faces and concurs to the abovementioned deficits, following a recursive trend.

The first pathway is thought to be linked to the second one, which concerns the Mirror Neuron System (MNs). In fact, the ability to extract salient information from faces has a relationship with the ability to adequately respond to the perceived emotion. Impairment at the level of the MNs involves impaired simulation processes, a lack of embodied empathy and poor reciprocal social abilities, including joint attention, gestural recognition and communication. MNs, in fact, allows to embody a "supramodal representation" of action, functioning as a bridge between seeing and doing (Williams, Whiten, Suddendorf, & Perrett, 2001).

The model also suggests a link between the second and the third pathway, in that the competencies related to the MNs have a strict connection to the development of ToM. In fact, both imitation and the attribution of mental states require the acquisition of others' perspective. Moreover, this is also assumed by one of the two principal models of how ToM operates, that is the Simulation Theory (Williams et al., 2001). Even if the amygdala has been described to have a role in mentalization processes (See Par. 4.3), the model proposes a more specific network for the attribution of mental states, emerging from consistent and influential neuroimaging evidences (Castelli et al., 2002). This network, defined as the "mentalizing network", includes the Medial Prefrontal Cortex (MPFC), the temporal poles and the Superior Temporal Sulcus, which are independent from task and modality.

The brain areas associated with the described pathways are supposed to be part of a more extensive and complex network and work together to process meaningful and useful information from faces, including perceptual (FFA), emotional (amygdala), cognitive (ToM) and mirroring processing. Emerging evidence with studies of a broader range of tasks showed disrupted brain connections in individuals with autism and suggested ASD to be an underconnectivity syndrome (Just, Cherkassky, Keller, & Minshew, 2004). In particular, the social deficit observed in autism may be due to underconnectivity among the mentalizing network (Path 3) (Castelli et al., 2002), and/or between emotional (amygdala) and perceptual (FFA) processing (Schultz, 2005), within the proposed Path 1 (Kana, Keller, Cherkassky, Minshew, & Just, 2009; Koshino et al., 2008).

Moreover, it has been shown that there is a weakened functional connectivity between anterior (MPFC) and posterior (FFA) brain areas (Kana et al., 2009; Koshino et al., 2008). These results have important implications to explain the relationship between mentalizing abilities and the particular ASD processing deficit. In fact, according to this hypothesis, ASD would use a more visually oriented approach to faces because of poor information transmission. According to our model, this could be interpreted as an inter-pathways underconnectivity, in particular between Path 1 and 3. This suggestion should be more extensively explored and integrated with regard to the role of the MNs for the underconnectivity theory, to ground on successive empirical evidence.

Impairment in at least one of the three pathways could lead to a compromised emotional facial expressions decoding in ASD. The size of the deficit could explain the severity within the autistic spectrum, which is characterized by quantitative more than qualitative differences. In the case of AS, for example, there could be a more circumscribed deficit which permits some useful compensatory strategies. Indeed, we suppose that, based on the type and deepness of pathway-related deficits, subjects could adopt specific compensatory strategies.

Common compensatory strategies may be found in preferential attention to parts rather than wholes (Shah & Frith, 1993); the recourse to linguistic components and structures specialized for verbal labeling (Baron-Cohen et al., 1999); a more visually oriented processing, together with the activation of areas involved in object processing (Koshino et al., 2008); social indirectness and avoidance (Schultz et al., 2003) and increased attention to external, more than internal information in responding to social cues (Kennedy & Courchesne, 2008).

Even if the presence of compensatory strategies was already proposed in the second version of the model, it still constitutes a peculiar feature of the present revised model, because now it can be more directly related to specific levels of impairment (based on specific functions) and preferential pathways.

To conclude, the model tries to describe and explain the impaired emotional facial decoding in ASD and AS. Furthermore, it could also be applied to the emotional domain in general, accounting for both emotion detection and expression, for both input and output abilities.

References

Aggleton, J. P. (1992). The amygdala: Neurobiological aspects of emotion, memory and mental dysfunction. New York, NY: *Wiley.*

Amenta, S., Ferrari, C., & Balconi, M. (2014). Facial expression decoding in autistic and Asperger children. In V. B. Patel, V. R. Preedy, & C. R. Martin (Eds.), *A comprehensive guide to autism*. London, UK: *Springer.*

American Psychiatric Association (1994). Diagnostic and statistical manual of mental disorders. 4th ed., Washington, DC: American Psychiatric Association.

American Psychiatric Association (2000). Diagnostic and statistical manual of mental disorders. 4th ed., Text Revision, Washington, DC: American Psychiatric Association.

American Psychiatric Association (2013). Diagnostic and statistical manual of mental disorders. 5th ed., Arlington, VA: *American Psychiatric Publishing.*

Asperger, H. (1991). Autistic psychopathy in childhood. In U. Frith (Ed. & Trans.), *Autism and Asperger's Syndrome* (pp. 37-92). Cambridge, UK: *Cambridge University Press.* (Original work published 1944).

Balconi, M. (2008). A theoretical overview on communicative, cognitive and neuropsychological correlates of facial expression recognition. In M. Balconi (Ed.), *Emotional face comprehension*. New York, NY: *Nova Science Publishers.*

Balconi, M., Amenta, S., & Ferrari, C. (2012). Emotional decoding in facial expression, scripts and videos: A comparison between normal, autistic and Asperger children. *Research in Autism Spectrum Disorder,* 6, 193-203.

Balconi, M., & Bortolotti, A. (2012). Detection of the facial expression of emotion and self-report measures in empathic situations are influenced by sensorimotor circuit inhibition by low-frequency rTMS. *Brain Stimulation,* 5(3), 330-336.

Balconi, M., & Bortolotti, A. (2013a). Emotional face recognition, empathic trait (BEES), and cortical contribution in response to positive and negative cues. The effect of rTMS on dorsal medial prefrontal cortex. *Cognitive Neurodynamics,* 7(1),13-21.

Balconi, M., Bortolotti, A., & Gonzaga, L. (2011). Emotional face recognition, EMG response, and medial prefrontal activity in empathic behavior. *Neuroscience Research,* 71(3), 251-259.

Balconi, M., & Canavesio, Y. (2013a). High-frequency rTMS improves facial mimicry and detection responses in an empathic emotional task. *Neuroscience,* 236,12-20.

Balconi, M., & Carrera, A. (2007). Emotional representation in facial expression and script. A comparison between normal and autistic children. *Research in Developmental Disabilities,* 28(4), 409-22.

Balconi, M., & Carrera, A. (2008). Facial emotion recognition impairment in autism. In M. Balconi (Ed.), *Emotional face comprehension: Neuropsychological perspectives* (pp. 155-204). New York, NY: *Nova Science Publishers.*

Balconi, M., & Carrera, A. (2011). Cross-modal integration of emotional face and voice in congruous and incongruous pairs: The P2 ERP effect. *Journal of Cognitive Psychology,* 23, 132-139.

Balconi, M., & Ferrari, C. (2012). Subliminal and supraliminal processing of facial expression of emotions: Brain oscillation in the left/right frontal area. *Brain Sciences,* 2, 85-100.

Balconi, M., & Pozzoli, U. (2003). Face-selective processing and the effect of pleasant and unpleasant emotional expressions on ERP correlates. *International Journal of Psychophysiology,* 49(1), 67-74.

Balconi, M., & Pozzoli, U. (2005). Morphed facial expressions elicited a N400 ERP effect: a domain-specific semantic module? *Scandinavian Journal of Psychology,* 46(6), 467-474.

Balconi, M., & Pozzoli, U. (2009). Arousal effect on emotional face comprehension: Frequency band changes indifferent time intervals. *Physiology & Behavior,* 97(3-4), 455-62.

Baron-Cohen, S. (1989a). Are autistic children behaviourists? An examination of their mental-physical and appearance-reality distinctions. *Journal of Autism and Developmental Disorders,* 19, 579-600.

Baron-Cohen, S. (1995). Mindblindness: An essay on autism and theory of mind. Cambridge, MA: *MIT Press.*

Baron-Cohen, S. (2002). The extreme male brain theory of autism. *Trends in Cognitive Sciences,* 6, 248-54.

Baron-Cohen, S., Leslie, A. M., & Frith, U. (1985). Does the autistic child have a "theory of mind"? *Cognition,* 1, 37-46.

Baron-Cohen, S., Ring, H. A., Bullmore, E.T., Wheelwright, S., Ashwin, C., & Williams, S. C. (2000). The amygdala theory of autism. *Neuroscience & Biobehavioral Reviews,* 24, 355-364.

Baron-Cohen, S., Ring, H.A., Wheelwright, S., Bullmore, E.T., Brammer, M., Simmons, A., & Williams, S. C. (1999). Social intelligence in the normal and autistic brain: An fMRI study. *European Journal of Neuroscience,* 11, 1891-1898.

Baron-Cohen, S., Spitz, A., & Cross, P. (1993). Do children with autism recognize surprise? A research note. *Cognition & Emotion,* 7, 507-516.

Bartlett, F. C. (1932). Remembering: A study in experimental and social psychology. Cambridge, UK: *Cambridge University Press.*

Beall, P. M., Moody, E. J., McIntosh, D. N., Hepburn, S. L., & Reed, C. L. (2008). Rapid facial reactions to emotional facial expressions in typically developing children and children with autism spectrum disorder. *Journal of Experimental Child Psychology,* 101, 206-223.

Bejerot, S. (2007). An autistic dimension: a proposed subtype of obsessive-compulsive disorder. *Autism,* 11, 101-110.

Bruce, V., & Young, A. (1998). A theoretical perspective for understanding brain recognition. In A. W. Young (Ed.), *Face and mind.* Oxford, UK: *Oxford University Press.*

Bushnell, I. W. (2001). Mother's face recognition in newborn infants: Learning and memory. *Infant and Child Development,* 10, 67-74.

Carey, S., & Diamond, R. (1994). Are faces perceived as configurations more by adults than by children? *Visual Cognition*, 1, 253-274.

Castelli, F., Frith, C.D., Happé, F., & Frith, U. (2002). Autism, Asperger syndrome and brain mechanisms for the attribution of mental states to animated shapes. *Brain,* 125(Pt 8), 1839-1849.

Celani, G., Battacchi, M. W., & Arcidiacono, L. (1999). The understanding of the emotional meaning of facial expressions in people with autism. *Journal of Autism and Developmental Disorders*, 29(1), 57-66.

Critchley, H. D. (2009). Psychophysiology of neural, cognitive and affective integration: fMRI and autonomic indicants. *International Journal of Psychophysiology*, 73, 88-94.

Critchley, H. D., Daly, E. M., Bullmore, E. T., Williams, S. C., Van Amelsvoort, T., Robertson, D. M., …Murphy, D. G. (2000). The functional neuroanatomy of social behavior: Changes in cerebral blood flow when people with autistic disorder process facial expressions. *Brain,* 123, 2203-2212.

Dapretto, M., Davies, M. S., Pfeifer, J. H., Scott, A. A., Sigman, M., & Bookheimer, S.Y. (2006). Understanding emotions in others: Mirror neuron dysfunction in children with autism spectrum disorders. *Nature Neuroscience,* 9(1), 28-30.

Davies, S., Bishop, D., Manstead, A. S. R., & Tantam, D. (1994). Face perception in children with autism and Asperger Syndrome. *Journal of Child Psychology and Psychiatry*, 35, 1033-1057.

Dawson, G., Webb, S. J., & McPartland, J. (2005). Understanding the nature of face processing impairment in autism: Insights from behavioral and electrophysiological studies. *Developmental Neuropsychology,* 7(3), 403-424.

Deeley, Q., Daly, E. M., Surguladze, S., Page, L., Toal, F., Robertson, D., …Murphy, D. G. (2007). An event related functional Magnetic Resonance Imaging study of facial emotion processing in Asperger Syndrome. *Biological Psychiatry,* 62, 207-217.

Denckla, M. (1983). The neuropsychology of social-emotional learning disabilities. *Archives of Neurology,* 40, 461-462.

Deruelle, C., Rondan, C., Gepner, B., & Tardif, C. (2004). Spatial frequency and face processing in children with autism and Asperger syndrome. *Journal of Autism and Developmental Disorders*, 34(2), 199-210.

Doi, H., Fujisawa, T. X., Kanai, C., Ohta, H., Yokoi, H., Iwanami, A., Shinohara, K. (2013). Recognition of facial expressions and prosodic cues with graded emotional intensities in adults with Asperger syndrome. *Journal of Autism and Developmental Disorders,* 43, 2099-2113.

Eimer, M. (2000). Effects of face inversion on the structural encoding and recognition of faces: Evidence from event-related brain potentials. *Cognitive Brain Research,* 10, 145-158.

Ekman, P. (1992). An argument for basic emotions. *Cognition and Emotion,* 6, 169-200.

Elgar, K., & Campbell, R. (2001). Annotation: The cognitive neuroscience of face recognition: Implications for developmental disorders. *The Journal of Child Psychology and Psychiatry and Allied Disciplines,* 42, 705-717.

Endo, N., Endo, M., Kirita, T., & Maruyama, K. (1992). The effects of expression on face recognition. *Tohoku Psychologica Folia*, 52, 37-44.

Field, T. M., Woodson, R., Greenberg, R., & Cohen, D.J. (1982). Discrimination and imitation of facial expressions by neonates. *Science,* 218, 179-181.

Fox, E., Russo, R., Bowles, R. J., & Dutton, K. (2001). Do threatening stimuli draw or hold visual attention in sub-clinical anxiety? *Journal of Experimental Psychology: General,* 130(4), 681-700.

Frith, C.D. (2003). What do imaging studies tell us about the neural basis of autism? *Novartis Foundation Symposium,* 251, 149-66.

Frith, U. (1989a). A new look at language and communication in autism [Review]. *British Journal of Disorders of Communication,* 24, 123-50.

Frith, U. (1989b). Autism: Explaining the enigma. Oxford, UK: *Basil Blackwell.*

Frith, U., & Frith, C. D. (2003). Development and neurophysiology of mentalizing. Philosophical Transactions of the Royal Society of London. Series B, *Biological Sciences,* 358(1431), 459-473.

Gallese, V. (2005). "Being-like-me": Self-other identity, mirror neurons, and empathy. In S. Hurley & N. Chater, (Eds.), *Perspectives on Imitation* (pp. 101-118). Cambridge, MA: *MIT Press.*

Ghaziuddin, M. (2010). Should the DSM-5 drop Asperger syndrome? *Journal of Autism and Developmental Disorders,* 40(9), 1146-1148.

Golarai, G., Grill-Spector, K., & Reiss, A. L. (2006). Autism and the development of face processing. *Clinical Neuroscience Research,* 6, 145-160.

Goren, C. C., Sarty, M., & Wu, P. Y. K. (1975). Visual following and pattern discrimination of face-like stimuli by newborn infants. *Pediatrics,* 56, 544-549.

Grelotti, D. J., Gauthier, I., & Schultz, R. T. (2002). Social interest and the development of cortical face specialization: What autism teaches us about face processing. *Developmental Psychobiology,* 40, 213-225.

Grelotti, D. J., Klin, A. J., Gauthier, I., Skudlarski, P., Cohen, D. J., Gore, J. C., ...Schultz, R. T. (2005). fMRI activation of the fusiform gyrus and amygdala to cartoon characters but not to faces in a boy with autism. *Neuropsychologia,* 43, 373-385.

Grice, S., Spratling, M., Karmiloff-Smith, A., Halit, H., Csibra, G., de Haan, M., & Johnson, M. H. (2001). Disordered visual processing and oscillatory brain activity in autism and Williams syndrome. *NeuroReport,* 12(12), 2697-2700.

Grossman, J. B., Klin, A., Carter, A. S., & Volkmar, F. R. (2000). Verbal bias in recognition of facial emotions in children with Asperger syndrome. *Journal of Child Psychology and Psychiatry and Allied Disciplines,* 41, 369-379.

Hadjikani, N. M., Joseph, R. M., Snyder, J., & Tager-Flusberg, H. (2006). Anatomical differences in the mirror neuron system and social cognition network in autism. *Cerebral Cortex,* 16, 1276-1312.

Hall, G. B. C., Szechtman, H., & Nahmias, C. (2003). Enhanced salience and emotion recognition in autism: a PET study. *American Journal of Psychiatry,* 160, 1439-1441.

Hamann, S. (2012). Mapping discrete and dimensional emotions onto the brain: Controversies and consensus. *Trends in Cognitive Sciences,*16(9), 458-466.

Hamilton, A. F. (2008). Emulation and mimicry for social interaction: A theoretical approach to imitation in autism. *Quarterly Journal of Experimental Psychology,* 61(1), 101-115.

Hanley, M., McPhillips, M., Mulhern, G., & Riby, D. M. (2013). Spontaneous attention to faces in Asperger syndrome using ecologically valid static stimuli. *Autism,* 17(6), 754-761.

Happé, F. (1996a). Studying weak central coherence at low levels: Children with autism do not succumb to visual illusions. A research note. *Journal of Child Psychology and Psychiatry,* 37(7), 873-877.

Happé, F., Ehlers, S., Fletcher, P., Frith, U., Johansson, M., Gillberg, C., ...*Frith, C.D.* (1996). "Theory of mind" in the brain. Evidence from a PET scan study of Asperger syndrome. *NeuroReport,* 8(1), 197-201.

Happé, F., & Frith, U. (1996). The neuropsychology of autism. *Brain,* 119, 1377-1400.

Hermans, E. J., Van Wingen, G., Bos, P. A., Putman, P., & Van Honk, J. (2009). Reduced spontaneous facial mimicry in women with autistic traits. *Biological Psychology,* 80, 348-353.

Hermelin, B., & O'Connor, N. (1967). Remembering of words by psychotic and subnormal children. *British Journal of Psychology,* 58, 213-218.

Horel, J. A., Keating, E. G., & Misantone, L. J. (1975). Partial Kluver-Bucy syndrome produced by destroying temporal neocortex or amygdala. *Brain Research,* 94, 347-359.

Howard, M. A., Cowell, P. E., Boucher, J., Broks, P., Mayes, A., Farrant, A., & Roberts, N. (2000). Convergent neuroanatomical and behavioral evidence of an amygdala hypothesis of autism. *NeuroReport,* 11, 2931-2935.

Humphreys, K., Minshew, N., Leonard, G. L., & Behrmann, M. (2007). A fine-grained analysis of facial expression processing in high-functioning adults with autism. *Neuropsychologia*, 45, 685-695.

Itier, R., & Taylor, M. (2002). Inversion and contrast polarity reversal affect both encoding and recognition processes of unfamiliar faces: A repetition study using ERPs. *NeuroImage,* 15, 353–372.

Jemel, B., Mottron, L., & Dawson, M. (2006). Impaired face processing in autism: Fact or artifact? *Journal of Autism and Developmental Disorders,* 36(1), 91-106.

Just, M. A., Cherkassky, V. L., Keller, T. A., & Minshew, N. J. (2004). Cortical activation and synchronization during sentence comprehension in high-functioning autism: evidence of underconnectivity. *Brain,* 127(8), 1811-1821.

Kamio, Y., Wolf, J., & Fein, D. (2006). Automatic processing of emotional faces in high-functioning pervasive developmental disorders: An affective priming study. *Journal of Autism and Developmental Disorders,* 36, 155-167.

Kana, R. K., Keller, T. A., Cherkassky, V. L., Minshew, N. J., & Just, M. A. (2009). Atypical frontal-posterior synchronization of Theory of Mind regions in autism during mental state attribution. *Social Neuroscience,* 4(2), 135-152.

Kätsyri, J., Saalasti, S., Tiippana, K., Von Wendt, L., & Sams, M. (2008). Impaired recognition of facial emotions from low-spatial frequencies in Asperger syndrome. *Neuropsychologia,* 46, 1888-1897.

Kennedy, D. P., & Courchesne, E. (2008). Functional abnormalities of the default network during self- and other-reflection in autism. *Social, Cognitive and Affective Neuroscience,* 3(2), 177-190.

Keysers, C., & Gazzola, V. (2006). Towards a unifying neural theory of social cognition. *Progress in Brain Research,* 156, 383-406.

Klin, A., Jones, W., Schultz, R., Volkmar, F.R., & Cohen, D.J. (2002). Visual fixation patterns during viewing of naturalistic social situations as predictors of social competence in individuals with autism. *Archives of General Psychiatry,* 59, 809-816.

Klin, A., McPartland, J., & Volkmar, F. R. (2005). Asperger syndrome. In: F. R. Volkmar, A. Klin, R. Paul, & D. J. Cohen (Eds), *Handbook of autism and pervasive developmental disorders* (pp. 88-125). Hoboken, NJ: *Wiley.*

Klin, A., & Volkmar, F. R. (1995). Asperger's Syndrome. Guidelines for assessment and diagnosis. M. D. Yale Child Study Center, New Haven, CT: *Learning Disabilities Association of America.*

Knobe, J. (2003). Intentional action in folk psychology: An experimental investigation. *Philosophical Psychology,* 16, 309-324.

Koshino, H., Kana, R. K., Keller, T. A., Cherkassky, V. L., Minshew, N. J., & Just, M. A. (2008). fMRI investigation of working memory for faces in autism: Visual coding and Underconnectivity with Frontal Areas. *Cerebral Cortex,* 18, 289-300.

Landa, R., Folstein, S. E., & Isaacs, C. (1991). Spontaneous narrative-discourse performance of parents of autistic individuals. *Journal of Speech and Hearing Disorders,* 34, 1339-1345.

Lang, P. J., Bradley, M. M., & Cuthbert, B. N. (1990). Emotion, attention, and the startle reflex. *Psychological Review,* 97, 377-395.

Law Smith, M. J., Montagne, B., Perrett, D. I., Gill, M., & Gallagher, L. (2010). Detecting subtle facial emotion recognition deficits in high-functioning Autism using dynamic stimuli of varying intensities. *Neuropsychologia,* 48, 2777–2781.

Leslie, A. (1991). The theory of mind impairment in autism: Evidence for a modular mechanisms of development? In A. Whiten, (Ed.), *Natural theories of mind.* Oxford, UK: *Basil Blackwell.*

Leslie, A. M., & Keeble, S. (1987). Do six-month-olds perceive causality? *Cognition,* 25, 265-288.

Leslie, A. M., & Roth, D. (1993). What Autism Teaches Us about Metarepresentation. In S. Baron-Cohen, H. Tager-Flusberg, & D.J. Cohen (Eds.), *Understanding Other Minds: Perspectives from Autism* (pp. 83-111). Oxford, UK: *University Press.*

Loveland, K. A., Tunali-Kotoski, B., Chen, Y. R., Brelsford, K. A., Ortegon, J., & Pearson, D. A. (1995). Intermodal perception of affect in persons with autism or Down syndrome. *Development and Psychopathology,* 7(3), 409-418.

Loveland, K. A., Tunali-Kotoski, B., Chen, Y. R., Ortegon, J., Pearson, D. A., Brelsford, K. A., & Gibbs, M. C. (1997). Emotion recognition in autism: Verbal and nonverbal information. *Development & Psychopathology,* 9(3), 579-593.

Lundquist, L. O., & Dimberg, A. (1995). Facial expressions are contagious. *Journal of Psychophysiology,* 9, 203-211.

Marcus, D. J., & Nelson, C. A. (2001). Neural basis and development of face recognition in autism. *CNS Spectrums,* 6, 36-59.

Marotta, A., Pasini, A., Ruggiero, S., Maccari, L., Rosa, C., Lupiáñez, J., & Casagrande M. (2013). Inhibition of Return in response to eye gaze and peripheral cues in young people with Asperger's Syndrome. *Journal of Autism and Developmental Disorders,* 43, 917-923.

Mathersul, D., McDonald, S., & Rushby, J.A. (2013a). Automatic facial responses to affective stimuli in high-functioning adults with autism spectrum disorder. *Physiology & Behavior,* 109, 14-22.

Mathersul, D., McDonald, S., & Rushby, J. A. (2013b). Autonomic arousal explains social cognitive abilities in high-functioning adults with autism spectrum disorder. *International Journal of Psychophysiology,* 89, 475-482.

McIntosh, D. N., Reichmann-Decker, A., Winkielman, P., & Wilbarger, J. L. (2006). When the social mirror breaks: Deficits in automatic, but not voluntary, mimicry of emotional facial expressions in autism. *Developmental Science,* 9, 295-302.

McPartland, J., Dawson, G., Webb, S., Panagiotides, H., & Carver, L. (2004). Event-related brain potentials reveal anomalies in temporal processing of faces in autism spectrum disorder. *Journal of Child Psychology and Psychiatry,* 45(7), 1235-1245.

McPartland, J., & Klin, A. (2006). Asperger's Syndrome. *Adolescent Medicine Clinics,* 17(3), 771-788.

Morris, J., Friston, K., Buchel, C., Frith, C. D., Young, A., Calder, A., & Dolan, R. J. (1998). A neuromodulatory role for the human amygdala in processing emotional facial expressions. *Brain,* 121, 47-57.

Newman, T. M., Macomber, D., Naples, A.J., Babitz, T., Volkmar, F.R., Grigorenko, E.L. (2007). Hyperlexia in children with autism spectrum disorders. *Journal of Autism and Developmental Disorders,* 37(4), 760-74.

Nishitani, N., Avikainen, S., & Hari, R. (2004). Abnormal imitation-related cortical activation sequences in Asperger's Syndrome. *Annals of Neurology,* 55, 558-562.

Oberman, L. M., Winkielman, P., & Ramachandran, V. S. (2009). Slow echo: Facial EMG evidence for the delay of spontaneous, but not voluntary, emotional mimicry in children with autism spectrum disorders. *Developmental Science,* 12, 510-520.

O'Connor, K., Hamm, J. P., & Kirk, I. J. (2007). Neurophysiological responses to face, facial regions and objects in adults with Asperger's Syndrome: An ERP investigation. *International Journal of Psychophysiology,* 63, 283-293.

Or, C. C., & Wilson, H. R. (2013). Implicit face prototype learning from geometric information. *Vision Research,* 82,1-12.

Pelphrey, K., Sasson, N., Reznick, S., Paul, G., Goldman, B., & Piven, J. (2002). Visual scanning of faces in autism. *Journal of Autism and Developmental Disorders,* 32(4), 249-261.

Posner, M. I. (1980). Orienting of attention. *Quarterly Journal of Experimental Psychology,* 32, 3-25.

Posner, M. I., & Cohen, Y. (1984). Components of visual orienting. In H. Bouma & D.G. Bouwhuis (Eds.), *Attention and performance X.* Hove, UK: Lawrence Erlbaum Associates Ltd.

Prior, M., Eisenmajer, R., Leekam, S., Wing, L., Gould, J., Ong, B., & Dowe, D. (1998). Are there subgroups within the autistic spectrum disorders? A cluster analysis of a group of children with autistic spectrum disorders. *Journal of child psychology and psychiatry,* 39(6), 893-902.

Ramachandran, V. S., & Oberman, L. M. (2006). Broken mirrors: A theory of autism. *Scientific American,* 295, 62-69.

Ro, T., Russell, C., & Lavie, N. (2001). Changing faces: A detection advantage in the flicker paradigm. *Psychological Science,* 12(1), 94-99.

Rogers, S. J., Hepburn, S. L., Stackhouse, T., & Wehner, E. (2003). Imitation performance in toddlers with autism and those with other developmental disorders. *Journal of Child Psychology and Psychiatry,* 44, 763-781.

Rourke, B. P. (1989). Nonverbal learning disabilities: The syndrome and the model. New York, NY: *The Guilford Press.*

Russell, J.A. (1980). A circumplex model of affect. *Journal of Personality and Social Psychology,* 39, 1161-1178.

Russell, J. A. (2003). Core affect and the psychological construction of emotion. *Psychological Review,* 110, 145-172.

Sasson, N. J., & Touchstone, E. W. (2014). Visual attention to competing social and object images by preschool children with Autism Spectrum Disorder. *Journal of Autism and Developmental Disorders*, 44, 584-592.

Schultz, R. T. (2005). Developmental deficits in social perception in autism: The role of the amygdala and fusiform face area. *International Journal of Developmental Neuroscience,* 23, 125-141.

Schultz, R. T., Grelotti, D. J., Klin, A., Kleinman, J., Van der Gaag, C., Marois, R., & Skudlarski, P. (2003). The role of the fusiform face area in social cognition: Implications for the pathobiology of autism. *Philosophical Transactions of the Royal Society of London. Series B: Biological Sciences*, 358, 415-427.

Shah, A., & Frith, U. (1993). Why do autistic individuals show superior performance on the block design task? *Journal of Child Psychology and Psychiatry,* 34, 1351-1364.

Smalley, S. L., & Asarnow, R. F. (1990). Cognitive subclinical markers in autism. *Journal of Autism and Developmental Disorders,* 20, 271-278.

Solso, R. L., & McCarthy, J. E. (1981). Prototype formation of faces: A case of pseudo-memory. *British Journal of Psychology,* 72, 499-503.

Stephens, C. L., Christie, I. C., & Friedman, B. H. (2010). Autonomic specificity of basic emotions: Evidence from pattern classification and cluster analysis. *Biological Psychology,* 84, 463-473.

Stone, W. L., Ousley, O. Y., & Littleford, C. L. (1997). Motor imitation in young children with autism: What's the object? *Journal of Abnormal Child Psychology*, 25, 475-485.

Surguladze, S. A., Brammer, M. J., Young, A. W., Andrew, A. T., Williams, S. C. R., & Phillips, M. L. (2003). A preferential increase in the extrastriate response to signals of danger. *Neuroimage,* 19, 1317-1328.

Tager-Flusberg, H. (1991). Semantic processing in the free recall of autistic children: Further evidence for a cognitive deficit. *British Journal of Psychology,* 9, 417-430.

Theeuwes, J., & Van der Stigchel, S. (2006). Faces capture attention: Evidence from inhibition of return. *Visual Cognition,* 13(6), 657-665.

Tranel, D., & Hyman, B. T. (1990). Neuropsychological correlates of bilateral amygdala damage. *Archives on Neurology,* 47, 349-355.

Voeller, K. K. S. (1986). Right hemisphere deficit syndrome in children. *American Journal of Psychiatry,* 143, 1004-1009.

Volkmar, F. R., & Klin, A. (2000). Diagnostic issues in Asperger syndrome. In: A. Klin, & F. R. Volkmar (Eds.), *Asperger syndrome* (pp. 25-71). New York, NY: *The Guilford Press.*

Vuilleumier, P., Richardson, M. P., Armony, J. L., Driver, J., & Dolan, R. J. (2004). Distant influences of amygdala lesion on visual cortical activation during emotional face processing. *Nature Neuroscience,* 7, 1271-1278.

Want, S. C., & Harris, P. L. (2001). Learning from other people's mistakes: Causal understanding in learning to use a tool. *Child Development,* 72, 431-443.

Weintraub, S., & Mesulam, M. M. (1983). Developmental learning disabilities of the right hemisphere. Emotional, interpersonal, and cognitive components. *Archives of Neurology*, 11, 463-468.

Williams, J. H. G., Whiten, A., Suddendorf, T., & Perrett, D. I. (2001). Imitation, mirror neurons and autism. *Neuroscience and Behavioral Reviews,* 25, 287-295.

Wing, L. (1981). Asperger's Syndrome: A clinical account. *Psychological Medicine*, 11, 115-129.

Wing, L., & Gould, J. (1979). Severe impairments of social interaction and associated abnormalities in children: Epidemiology and classification. *Journal of Autism and Developmental Disorders*, 9, 11-29.

Wolff, S., & Chick, J. (1980). Schizoid personality in childhood: a controlled follow-up study. *Psychological Medicine,* 10, 85-100.

Woodbury-Smith, M. R., & Volkmar, F. R. (2009). Asperger syndrome. *European Child & Adolescent Psychiatry,* 18(1), 2-11.

Yang, H. H., Savostyanov, A. N., Tsai, A. C., & Liou, M. (2011). Face recognition in Asperger syndrome: A study on EEG spectral power changes. *Neuroscience Letters*, 492, 84-88.

Young, A. W., Rowland, D., Calder, A. J., Etcoff, N. L., Seth, A., & Perrett, D. I. (1997). Facial expression megamix: Tests of dimensional and category accounts of emotion recognition. *Cognition,* 63(3), 271-313.

Zalla, T., & Leboyer, M. (2011). Judgment of intentionality and moral evaluation in individuals with high functioning autism. *Review of Philosophy and Psychology,* 2(4), 681-698.

Zalla, T., Sav, A. M., Stopin, A., Ahade, S., & Leboyer, M. (2009). Faux pas detection and intentional action in Asperger Syndrome. A replication on a French sample. *Journal of Autism and Developmental Disorder,* 39(2), 373-382.

In: Asperger Syndrome
Editor: Michael F. Shaughnessy
ISBN: 978-1-63463-810-4

Chapter 9

Communicative Behavior of Speakers with Asperger Syndrome from the Quick Protocol for Pragmatic Assessment (QPPA)

Francisco J. Rodríguez Muñoz*
University of Almería, Spain

Abstract

From the Quick Protocol for Pragmatic Assessment (QPPA), the communicative behavior of 20 speakers with Asperger Syndrome (AS) was assessed. The scale was composed of 17 items that were grouped in two ways: (i) general, specific, and grammar-based pragmatic abilities, and (ii) enunciative, textual, and interactive pragmatic abilities. Different pragmatic categories were associated with each of these dimensions in order to establish behavioral indicators that were altered from a communicative point of view. The most significant results suggest that items related to interactive and enunciative pragmatics, that exalt reception and expression processes, showed lower scores than those which were linked to textual areas, composition mechanisms. Finally, four levels of severity were taken into account for the classification of pragmatic deficits in the communicative behavior of people with AS.

Keywords: Communicative behavior, oral speech, pragmatic assessment

---

* Department Building n. 1 (Building A). Floor 2, Room 26. Ctra. Sacramento s/n, La Cañada de San Urbano, Almería, 04120, Spain. Email: frodriguez@ual.es. This research is part of the project "Ampliación y adaptación del corpus PERLA de datos clínicos en el marco del proyecto internacional Childes/Talkbank: perfiles pragmáticos y propuestas de intervención" (FFI2012-39325-C03-01), funded by the Ministry of Economy and Competitiveness (Government of Spain).

Introduction

In the last quarter of the twentieth century, research on language development adopted a new perspective defined by a communicative transition [1]; that is, the idea that language cannot be isolated from conversational contexts. The growing interest in evaluating the use of language using scientific methods based on observation has been marked by the emergence of various instruments that have allowed assessment of linguistic components from two basic perspectives: communication effectiveness and pragmatics.

In the first place, among the most useful tools that have appeared during recent decades for evaluating communication effectiveness, Gallardo [2] points out: ASHA FACS (Functional Assessment of Communication Skills) [3]; RICE (RIC Evaluation of Communication Problems in Right Hemisphere Dysfunction) [4]; ACE 6-11 (Assessment of Comprehension and Expression 6-11) [5]; CCC (Children's Communication Checklist) [6]; FCP-R (Functional Communication Profile-Revised) [7]; and CIM (Communication Independence Model) [8, 9].

In the second place, the main profiles that have focused on pragmatics have been: TOPL (Test Of Pragmatic Language) [10]; QCB (Quantification of Conversacional Behaviors) [11]; ACA (Activity Based Communication Approach) [12]; PPECC (Pragmatics Profile of Everyday Communication Skills in Children) [13]; PPECA (Pragmatics Profile of Everyday Communication Skills in Adults) [14]; PPCI (Profile of Pragmatic Impairment in Communication) [15]; BLOC (Batería de Lenguaje Objetiva y Criterial) [16]; CAPPA (Conversational Analysis Profile for People with Aphasia) [17]; CAPCCI (Conversation Analysis Profile for People with Cognitive Impairment) [18]; CCC (Children's Communication Checklist) [19]; PB (Pragmatic Battery) [20]; PELC-HD (Protocolo de Evaluación de Funciones Lingüísticas y Comunicativas para Pacientes de Hemisferio Derecho) [21]; and, more recently, PREP [QPPA] (Protocolo Rápido de Evaluación Pragmática [Quick Protocol for Pragmatic Assessment]) [2, 22, 23].

Quick Protocol for Pragmatic Assessment (QPPA)

Initially called PerLA Pragmatic Assessment Profile [2, 24], this battery includes a number of pragmatic categories that can provide guidance for the evaluation of possible communicative deficits in spontaneous spoken language. The Quick Protocol for Pragmatic Assessment (QPPA) emerged as a simplification of the previous profile, based on the reformulation of statements, and seeks greater clarity in the descriptive categories that compose it. Therefore, it has become a fast scan tool for professionals who are not necessarily specialists in linguistics [22]. For Gallardo [23], there are three pragmatic levels that account for the entire set of elements that are involved in dialogic oral interactions; that is, those communicative situations involving more than one interlocutor, preferably more than two: (i) enunciative pragmatics, where perception is oriented to the addresser, (ii) textual pragmatics, which is based on text construction, and (iii) interactive pragmatics, which relates to the addressee.

The *QPPA* adopts a broad conception of pragmatics since the protocol indirectly includes categories that involve grammatical components that may be affected in oral speech. Thus, the test distinguishes between a specific pragmatic ability, which does without lexical and morphosyntactic properties of discourse, and a grammar-based pragmatic ability, which embraces such units. It should also be noted that pragmatic alterations are hardly isolable, and measurable categories should reflect the close involvement among the different linguistic levels.

Table 1. Quick Protocol for Pragmatic Assessment (QPPA)

Appropriate Usage			
Assessment	Yes	No	Non-assessable
ENUNCIATIVE LEVEL			
1. Speech Acts			
1.1. Locutionary Speech Acts			
1.2. Propositional Speech Acts			
1.3. Use of pauses			
2. Editing Tasks			
2.1. Compensatory Locutionary Acts			
2.2. Compensatory Non-Verbal Acts			
2.3. Draft Acts			
3. Illocutionary Speech Acts			
4. Self-Repair			
5. Lexicalized Tropic Inference (Idioms)			
6. Cooperative Principle and Conversational Maxims			
6.1. Maxim of Quality			
6.2. Maxim of Quantity			
6.3. Maxim of Manner			
6.4. Maxim of Relevance			
6.5. Particularized Implicatures			
TEXTUAL LEVEL			
7. Textual Coherence: Superestructures			
8. Textual Coherence: Topic Management			
9. Lexical and Semantic Cohesion			
10. Morphological Cohesion			
11. Syntactic Cohesion			
INTERACTIVE LEVEL			
12. Turn Taking Agility			
13. Conversational Participation Index			
14. Predictability			
15. Gesture			
16. Gaze			
17. Priority			

In the QPPA, items 3–7 (except 6.3) and 11–15 refer to so-called specific pragmatic ability, items 1, 2, 6.3, and 8–10 pay attention to grammar-based pragmatic ability, and, finally, items 16 and 17 are included in order to assess a general ability, which combines the twenty-five items and sub-items that make up the scale. For the numerical measurement, only affirmative responses ('yes'), which are divided into the number of evaluated items ('yes' +

'no') without counting those that cannot be observed ('non-assessable'), are taken into account. Once the count value is obtained, it is multiplied by 100 for each of the listed factors: general ability, specific pragmatic ability, and grammar-based ability. However, besides the three previous indexes, as shown in Table 1, the *QPPA* allows us to turn our attention to the three pragmatic dimensions into which the scale may also be organized: enunciative (items 1-6), textual (items 7-11), and interactive pragmatics (items 12-17).

The three categories that enunciative pragmatics incorporates are speech acts, editing tasks (compensations), and inferential meanings. This last category is derived from observation of the cooperative principle and its conversational maxims. Locutionary speech acts (1.1) are negatively evaluated when the speaker presents alterations related to oral articulation, sound modulation, rhythm, and/or intonation. Each of these alterations can affect an utterance's verbal production. Propositional speech acts (1.2), however, allude to the problems of lexical access (e.g., anomia problems, a common symptom among aphasic patients). The third sub-item, the use of pauses (1.3), is assessed as negative when silences are abnormal or unexpected.

Editing tasks (item 2) [11] refer to the attempts made by the impaired speakers to compensate for their linguistic problems through exclamations, marked intonations, single syllables, words with vague meaning (2.1 compensatory locutionary acts), nonverbal gestures and actions, or circumlocutions or questions like "huh?" (2.3 draft acts). It should be noted that when items 1.1, 1.2, and 1.3 are positively scored, item 2 must not be evaluated since it is designed to assess the ability of those speakers who have severe difficulties expressing themselves verbally. Item 3, illocutionary speech acts, assesses the illocutionary force or the correspondence between what is intended to be communicated (intentionality) and what the speaker finally expresses. Item 4, self-repair, pays attention to the capacity for self-correction during the oral interaction. Item 5, lexicalized tropic inference, refers to idiom comprehension and production. Item 6 judges if communicative behaviors adapt to the cooperative principle [25], which is divided into four conversational maxims: (6.1) quality, the truthfulness of the provided information; (6.2) quantity, the excess or lack of information; (6.3) manner, clarity, non-ambiguity and orderliness; and (6.4) relevance, appropriateness of contributions in relation to the topic being developed in the conversation. The use of (6.5) particularized implicatures arises from the violation of maxims when speakers are aware of the violation and, for example, produce metaphorical, hyperbolic, or ironic expressions that depend on their own creativity.

Items 7 and 8 are related to a basic property, such as textual coherence, for which we can distinguish two levels: superstructures and topic management. The first level relates to the form of the discourse genre (narration, argumentation, exposition, description, dialogue); that is, the scheme that speakers have in mind and follow when they organize their discourse into different parts. The second level is highly linked to the maxim of relevance and is positively assessed when speakers contribute to the progress of the conversation by providing significant information.

Cohesion is distributed in three items: (9) lexical-semantic, (10) morphological, and (11) syntactic. The lexical-semantic cohesion is positively marked when co-referential mechanisms, such as pronominalization or lexical substitution, are adequately performed by speakers. Morphological cohesion (agrammatism) assesses irregularities in the use of grammatical morphemes; for example, it is negatively marked when words are built in an incomplete way. Syntactic cohesion (paragrammatism) is defined by violations in the construction of sentences, for example, improperly using the fundamental constituents of a syntactic structure. Item 12 refers to turn taking agility or the number of turns per minute. Item 13 deals with the conversational participation index; here, we ask whether the speaker's cooperation is proportional to that of the other participants. Item 14 considers predictability, which is positively assessed when there is a balance between reactive and predictive turns or between questions and answers.

With respect to non-verbal communication, item 15 includes gestures, which are assessed from the naturalness of the movements and facial expressions, as necessary complements of verbal behavior. Item 16 observes another non-verbal indicator, gaze. Item 16 reports on various aspects such as active listening, the request to participate in conversation or the change of turn. Item 17 is dedicated to priority and adequacy; when we talk about sociolinguistic adequacy, we are referring to the linguistic principle through which speakers adapt their speech to a particular context, more or less formal, and to their interlocutors. In other words, this criterion includes all that relates to the stylistic or functional variations of language, for example, the sociocultural principles of politeness and courtesy.

This diversity of categories, as Penn [26] indicates, is necessary because pragmatic units cannot be classified with the same methodological rigor that other language components allow and, once again, pragmatics adopts a multidimensional approach. Thus, the purpose of our pragmatic scale is to explore a wide range of behaviors that occur simultaneously during communicative exchanges.

Methods

Participants

The first step of our research consisted of the application of the *QPPA* in a population of 20 speakers with AS diagnosis. The clinical diagnosis of AS was validated by the psychologists who assisted in data collection and used the Social Communication Questionnaire (SCQ) [27] to confirm the presence of an autism spectrum disorder. With their parents' written informed consent, participants were videotaped for later analysis. 14 subjects with AS were from Asturias, Spain, while the other six came from Valencia, Spain. Data were collected in a person-to-person way in both geographic areas thanks to the collaboration of the Asturias Asperger Association and the Valencia Asperger Association. The chronologic age of the patients with AS was between 6 and 15 (M = 11.15); nineteen of them were male and we only counted one recording belonging to a Valencian female. At the moment of data collection, participants were not under any pharmacological treatment.

Materials

In order to collect oral data, we designed a graphic support for pragmatic training. The purpose of this instrument was to motivate a semi-oriented and inducted discourse with our participants based on picture description tasks. The support was composed of six illustrated cards with specific contents and independent questions. Thus, the function of the images was the same as a conversational script.

Procedure

The sample was taken in diverse multi-use rooms located at the Asturias Asperger Association and the Valencia Asperger Association. Before the recordings of the designed tasks in the graphic support, we provided the following general instructions to participants:

> I am going to show you six illustrated cards, and I will pose different questions to you about what you see in each picture. For example, I will ask you to put yourself in the place of some characters or to tell me a short story from the drawings. Please try to refer always to the card number.

We then showed participants each illustrated card and posed the questions that were to be answered orally.

Measurements

The annotations for the pragmatic assessment were completed on three different occasions for each participant: (i) after the videotaped interactions and before their transcription, (ii) after the transcription of oral data and before its revision, and (iii) in a final revision process.

For this purpose, we tried to determine a pragmatic profile of speakers with AS that offers relevant information about their communicative (verbal and nonverbal) behavior. Therefore, we calculated average values in the two directions that the scale allows: (i) pragmatic abilities grouped into general, specific, and grammar-based abilities and (ii) pragmatic dimensions grouped into enunciative, textual and interactive.

Pragmatic Profile of Speakers with AS

After having applied the QPPA to our 20 speakers with AS, the means for each subtype of ability were: (i) general pragmatic ability (76.5%), (ii) specific pragmatic ability (75.8%), and (iii) grammar-based ability (79.2%). According to the scores, pragmatic ability that includes grammatical constraints revealed the best result (thus, there were not remarkable deficits) and percentages corresponding to specific and general pragmatic skills were very close (we did not find significant deficits in these communicative spheres).

Table 2 shows the positive, negative, and non-assessable observations for the three dimensions that the pragmatic battery distinguishes for the whole sample of speakers with AS.

According to the above scores, pragmatic-textual ability revealed the best result (95%), followed by pragmatic-enunciative ability (79%) and, finally, pragmatic-interactive ability, which reflected the most deficient development (58%). More specifically, the percentage of participants who showed an appropriate use of each communicative behavior was distributed as follows in Table 3: locutionary speech acts (15%); propositional speech acts (65%); use of pauses (15%); compensatory locutionary acts (100%); compensatory non-verbal acts (45%); draft acts (100%); illocutionary speech acts (100%); self-repair (100%); lexicalized tropic inference (idioms) (30%); maxim of quality (90%); maxim of quantity (55%); maxim of manner (75%); maxim of relevance (80%); particularized implicatures (5%); textual coherence: superstructures (90%); textual coherence: topic management (85%); lexical and semantic cohesion (100%); morphological cohesion (100%); syntactic cohesion (100%); turn taking agility (75%); conversational participation index (55%); predictability (40%); gesture (35%); gaze (60%); and priority (80%). As shown in Table 3, we can sort the previous pragmatic deficits in AS according to four levels of severity.

Table 2. QPPA results according to enunciative, textual and interactive pragmatics

Enunciative pragmatics		Textual pragmatics		Interactive pragmatics	
Observation	*Total*	*Observation*	*Total*	*Observation*	*Total*
Positive	196	Positive	95	Positive	69
Negative	51	Negative	5	Negative	51
Non-assessable	33	Non-assessable	0	Non-assessable	0
TOTAL[a]	21%	TOTAL[a]	5%	TOTAL[a]	42%

a. Degree of pragmatic impairment.

Table 3. Levels of severity for each pragmatic deficit

Level of severity	Pragmatic deficit
Mild (0-25%)	compensatory locutionary acts; draft acts; illocutionary speech acts; self-repair; maxim of quality; maxim of manner; maxim of relevance; textual coherence: superstructures; textual coherence: topic management; lexical and semantic cohesion; morphological cohesion; syntactic cohesion; turn taking agility; priority.
Moderate (25-50%)	propositional speech acts; maxim of quantity; conversational participation index; gaze.
Severe (50-75%)	compensatory non-verbal acts; lexicalized tropic inference (idioms); predictability; gesture.
Profound (75-100%)	locutionary speech acts; use of pauses; particularized implicatures.

Conclusion

The quantitative analysis of data obtained from the QPPA has allowed us to interpret the results of the AS speakers' communicative behavior in two directions: (i) the assessment of general, specific, and grammar-based pragmatic abilities and (ii) the assessment of enunciative, textual, and interactive pragmatic abilities.

In the first case, there were no statistically significant differences between the percentages for specific (75.8%), grammar-based (79.2%), and general pragmatic abilities (76.5%). We did not find the same when comparing the three pragmatic spheres described by Gallardo [28]. Here, we observed a clear deficit in the interactive domain (58%), followed by a more acceptable score in the enunciative dimension (79%). Finally, the AS speakers did not show any important alteration in relation to textual pragmatics (95%). These data agree with previous research on pragmatic awareness in adults with AS [29].

According to the lines suggested by the *QPPA* in our 20 speakers with AS, it would be advisable to pay close attention to the pragmatic categories that the interactive dimension incorporates as they are significantly altered. However, we think that it would be unwise to avoid other categories linked to enunciative and textual pragmatics since, after a thorough analysis, these domains could reveal results different than expected.

References

[1] Díez-Itza, E. (1992). *Adquisición del lenguaje*. Oviedo: Pentalfa.

[2] Gallardo, B. (2007). *Pragmática para logopedas*. Cádiz: Universidad de Cádiz.

[3] Frattali, C. M., Thompson, C. M., Holland, A. L., Wohl, C. B., & Ferketic, M. M. (1995). *ASHA Functional Assessment of Communication Skills (FACS)*. Rockville, MD: American Speech-Language-Hearing Association.

[4] Halper, A. S., Cherney, L. R., Burns, M. S., & Mogil, S. I. (1996). RIC evaluation of communication problems in right hemisphere dysfunction-Revised (RICE-R). Test and administration manual. In A. S. Halper, L. R. Cherney, & M. S. Burns (Eds.), *Clinical Management of Right Hemisphere Dysfunction* (Second Edition, pp. 99-132). Gaithersburg, MD: Aspen Publishers Inc.

[5] Adams, C., Cooke, R., Crutchley, A., Hesketh, A., & Reeves, D. (2001). *Assessment of comprehension and expression 6-11*. Windsor: NFER-Nelson.

[6] Bishop, D. V. M., & Baird, G. (2001). Parent and teacher report of pragmatic aspects of communication: use of the children's communication checklist in a clinical setting. *Developmental Medicine and Child Neurology, 43* (12), 809-818.

[7] Kleiman, L. I. (2003). *Functional Communication Profile-Revised (FCP-R)*. East Moline, IL: Linguisystems.

[8] Gillette, Y. (2003). *Achieving communication independence: A comprehensive guide to assessment and intervention*. Eau Claire, WI: Thinking Publications.

[9] Gillette, Y. (2005). A communication independence model: guiding assessment and intervention with people who have severe communication disabilities and those who use AAC [E-text type]. http://www.speechpathology.com/articles/ article_detail.asp? article_id=215.

[10] Phelps-Terasaki, D., & Phelps-Gunn, T. (1992). *Test of Pragmatic Language*. East Moline, IL: Linguisystems.

[11] Crockford, C., & Lesser, R. (1994). Assessing functional communication in aphasia: clinical utility and time demands of three methods. *European Journal of Disorders of Communication, 29* (2), 165-182.

[12] Ahlsén, E. (1995). Pragmatics and aphasia. An activity based approach. *Gothenburg Papers in Theoretical Linguistics* (Monograph 77). Sweden: University of Gothenburg, Department of Linguistics.

[13] Dewart, H., & Summers, S. (1995). *The pragmatics profile of everyday communication skills in children*. Windsor: NFER-Nelson.

[14] Dewart, H., & Summers, S. (1996). *The pragmatics profile of everyday communication skills in adults*. Windsor: NFER-Nelson.

[15] Linscott, R. J., Knight, R. G., & Godfrey, H. (1996). The profile of functional impairment in communication (PFIC): A measure of communication impairment for clinical use. *Brain Injury, 10* (6), 397-412.

[16] Puyuelo, M., Wiig, E. H., Renom, J., & Solanas, A. (1997). *BLOC. Batería de Lenguaje Objetiva y Criterial*. Barcelona: Masson.

[17] Whitworth, A., Perkins, L., & Lesser, R. (1997). *Conversational Analysis Profile for People with Aphasia*. London: Whurr Pub.

[18] Whitworth, A., Perkins, L., & Lesser, R. (1997). *Conversational Analysis Profile for People with Cognitive Impairment*. London: Whurr Pub.

[19] Bishop, D. V. M. (1998). Development of the Children's Communication Checklist (CCC): A method for assessing qualitative aspects of communication impairment in children. *Journal of Child Psychology and Psychiatry, 39* (6), 879-891.

[20] Kasher, A., Batori, G., Soroker, N., Graves, D., & Zaidel, E. (1999). Effects on right- and left-hemisfere damage on uniderstanding conversational implicatures. *Brain Language, 68* (3), 566-590.

[21] Labos, E., Zabala, K., Atlasovich, C., Pavón, H., & Ferreiro, J. (2003). Evaluación de funciones lingüísticas y comunicativas en pacientes con lesión de hemisferio derecho. *Revista Neurológica Argentina, 28* (2), 96-103.

[22] Gallardo, B. (2008). Pragmática textual y TDAH. En *Actas del XXVI Congreso Internacional AELFA* (pp. 1-24) [E-text type]. http://www.uv.es/pauls/2008. GALLARDO.PragmatTextualTDAH.pdf.

[23] Gallardo, B. (2009). Valoración del componente pragmático a partir de datos orales. *Revista de neurología, 48* (Suppl. 2), S57-S61.

[24] Gallardo, B. (2006). Más allá de las palabras y su estructura: las categorías del componente pragmático. In E. Garayzábal (Ed.), *Lingüística clínica y logopedia* (pp. 81-196). Madrid: Antonio Machado Libros.

[25] Grice, H. P. (1975). Logic and conversation. In P. Cole, & J. L. Morgan (Eds.), *Syntax and Semantics: Volume 3. Speech Acts* (pp. 41-58). New York: Academic Press.

[26] Penn, C. (1999). Pragmatic assessment and therapy for persons with brain damage: what have clinicians gleaned in two decades? *Brain and Language, 68* (3), 535-552.

[27] Rutter, M., Bailey, A., & Lord, C. (2003). *The Social Communication Questionnaire*. Los Angeles, CA: Western Psychological Services.

[28] Gallardo, B. (2005). Categorías inferenciales en pragmática clínica. *Revista de neurología, 41* (Suppl. 1), 65-71.

[29] Rodríguez-Muñoz, F. J. (2012). La conciencia pragmática de adultos con síndrome de Asperger. *Revista de Logopedia, Foniatría y Audiología, 32* (1), 21-31.

Reviewed by Dra. Carmen Santos, New University of Lisbon, Portugal.
Reviewed by Dra. Susana Ridao Rodrigo, University of Murcia, Spain.

In: Asperger Syndrome
Editor: Michael F. Shaughnessy

ISBN: 978-1-63463-810-4

Chapter 10

Managing Asperger Syndrome in the Regular Classroom

Diane Montgomery*
Middlesex University, London, UK

Abstract

This chapter considers the characteristics and management of children with Asperger Syndrome within an educational context. Biographical details of referred cases are recorded and a clinical-educational picture of needs is drawn up. Parents and teachers are then involved in the proposed interventions as appropriate to enable the child to function in the regular classroom.

Keywords: Asperger, dual exceptionality, case analysis, regular classrooms, interventions

Introduction

Kanner in 1943 first identified Autism as a separate clinical condition in children. He distinguished it from childhood schizophrenia and other childhood psychoses. In 1944, Asperger (1979) identified a separate but seemingly autistic group with higher intellectual potential and less severe disabilities. He chose the name 'autistic psychopathy' to denote abnormality of personality but later the more neutral term of Asperger's Syndrome was used and now Asperger Syndrome (AS).

In the 1960s in London a clinical research group developed that pursued studies into these disorders and one of its leaders had an autistic child. In 1981 the Autistic Spectrum of Disorders (ASD) was identified by Lorna Wing to encompass the ever-widening group who had some aspects of the autistic condition. At that time educational provision for children

* Corresponding author: Professor Diane Montgomery, Learning Difficulties Research Project, 21, Butt Lane, Maldon, Essex, CM9 5HD, United Kingdom; email: dmont507@aol.com www.ldrp.org.uk

with ASD was being developed in special schools and special units in the UK. They dealt with those with the severest difficulties and it was not until the 1990s that the needs of children with AS began to be of concern in regular classrooms.

Before the introduction of the UK National Curriculum in 1991 with its detailed content and requirements for more formal teaching methods many primary schools could encompass the needs of children with AS and tolerate their more egocentric behaviours. Secondary schools tended to be less successful because of their constantly changing routines, different subjects, different teachers, changing teaching rooms and large crowds of unfamiliar people and pupils. There were also more pupils with AS in these settings and more likelihood of them being categorised and excluded as children with conduct disorders. These would finish up in PRUs (Pupil Referral Units) for assessment or special schools for children with Emotional and Behavioural Difficulties (EBD). In such settings those with AS were likely to learn more unsocial behaviours and be very prone to bullying.

Children with AS should receive a *Statement of Special Need* (DfEE, 2001) to secure extra funding for their social and communication needs. These could be met in regular classrooms if teachers were supported and better informed through Continuing Professional Development (CPD). By 2005 these programmes were well under way on a wide scale in the UK.

The American Psychological Association Diagnostic Manual DSM-V (2006) identified Autism Spectrum Disorders (ASD) as Pervasive Developmental Disorders (PDD). The condition known as Asperger Syndrome was included as ASD, High Functioning Autism (HFD) or PDD-NOS (PDD –Not Otherwise Specified). Autism and Asperger are the most similar and prevalent of the Autism Spectrum Disorders with an incidence of 1 per cent. They share many characteristics so that some argue they are varieties of the same underlying condition on a continuum from mild and moderate to severe and profound. Asperger cases would be at the upper more able end of this continuum but no precise cut-off points can as yet be determined. The condition also appears to shade off into the ‘eccentric normal’ range.

ASD is associated with a triad of impairments affecting social interaction, social communication and imagination (Wing 1981, 1996, 2008). It is most frequently accompanied by a limited, narrow, repetitive pattern of behaviour. It is the problem behaviours and poor social skills that teachers find most difficulty in managing.

Thus far there seems to be no single best fix intervention that can be applied to all children with Asperger Syndrome. Their different personalities, home circumstances, experiences, learning histories and abilities make it important for interventions to be more personalized. In addition it will be suggested that as part of the complexity it is often the school itself or the pedagogy that needs some modification to create an ‘Asperger friendly environment’. These issues, cases and relevant strategies will be discussed and exemplified in this chapter.

Method

Case study is the method used in this research to help understand the specific Asperger condition and how it may be alleviated. Each case has been given a pseudonym and was referred to the researcher by a parent or teacher for a second opinion unless otherwise specified. The need for a second opinion arose because the child had been given a Statement of Special Need (this involves diagnosis by a psychologist in consultation with other relevant professionals and input from the parents). The referrals arose because of concern about the validity of the original diagnosis and/or need to develop a more appropriate intervention plan.

Table 1. The Triad of Impairments

• **Social interaction**	difficulty with social relationships, e.g. appearing aloof and indifferent to other people, failure to follow social rules
• **Social communication**	difficulty with verbal and non-verbal communication, e.g. not really understanding the meaning of gestures, facial expressions or tone of voice
• **Imagination**	difficulty in the development of play and imagination, e.g. having a limited range of imaginative activities, possibly copied and pursued rigidly and repeatedly. Literal comprehension.

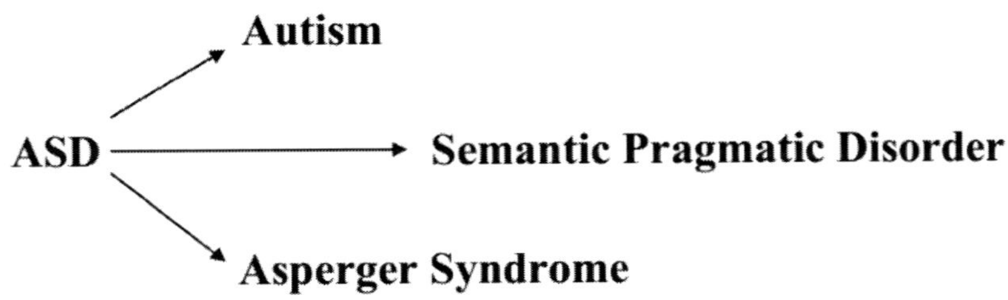

Semantic Pragmatic Disorder

SPD is identified as a separate condition (Bishop, 1989) on the ASD continuum in which social and behavioural skills and abilities are not markedly deficient. Dehaney (2000) identified the following features of the condition and they also apply in AS.

- Speech is fluent but lacks content and direction
- Explanations and answers to questions are not specific
- Comprehension is poor, particularly of abstract concepts understanding is often literal
- Interactive and imaginative play is poorly developed
- There is difficulty in recognising and expressing emotion
- Difficulty following the unwritten rules of conversation such as turn -taking, appropriateness and nonverbal language
- Weak temporal concepts causing confusion in school routines and chronological events
- Auditory memory is poor but rote learning is often a strength

- Poor attention skills, erratic motivation and distractibility
- Rarely asks for help or seeks clarification
- Behaviour is naive or eccentric
- Mechanical reading skills are good but comprehension is limited
- Self-esteem is low as a result of the problems and the difficulties caused by them. pp. 36-7

Dehaney concluded that in the current methods for teaching English and the 'literacy hour' (DfEE, 1998) the pace was too fast and the emphasis on oral and listening skills meant there was a failure to comprehend before the lesson moved on. Even simple stories required imagination or seeing things as others do and this was beyond these children. It was assumed that they could catch up what they miss but this was not possible. They needed special learning support and more strategies tailored to their needs.

Rutter (2005) found that a faulty gene transmitted ASD. But it can also be found in children and adults with pre-peri-and post-natal conditions such as anoxia at birth or specific viral conditions in infancy. This was true of fifty per cent of Wing's (1981) cases. There was no evidence that emotional problems and abnormal child rearing caused it and no specific organic pathology was implicated.

By 2009 understanding and knowledge of ASD had grown to such an extent that it was noted in *The Psychologist*, the official newsletter of the British Psychological Society, that autistic type behaviours were in fact common in a wide range of the 'normal' population.

Comorbidity

Comorbidity and therefore dual diagnosis has now been recognised in APA DSM-V (2006) so that an individual with AS may also be diagnosed with ADHD or other disorder. Rommelse et al. (2010) found that 30 to 80% of those with ASD had co-occurring symptoms of ADHD and 20 to 50% of individuals with ADHD also met the criteria for ASD.

ASD and ADHD are both developmental disorders in that they begin in childhood and often persist throughout life. They both occur more frequently in males than females. They occur in individuals with any level of IQ and can affect social functioning but their behavioural characteristics are distinct. ASD is characterised by impairments in social communication, imagination and restricted, repetitive behaviours and routines whereas ADHD is characterised by impulsivity, hyperactivity and inattention.

Twin studies show that these two conditions are highly heritable because they share a common genetic pathway (Ronald, 2014). It means that a parent having one child or partner with one condition is likely to have an increased chance of producing future children with either condition.

Neither ASD nor ADHD are 100% heritable and environmental risk conditions also operate. It is known that smoking during pregnancy is a risk factor for ADHD in offspring but not in ASD. In ASD a risk factor is higher paternal age but not for ADHD (Gabis et al. 2010). ASD and ADHD need to be regarded not as single construct disorders but co-occurring conditions so treatment interventions can be more appropriately refined.

It appears that the three different characteristics in ASD are caused by distinct genetic and environmental causes (Ronald 2014) called the 'fractionable autism triad' hypothesis (Happe et al. 2006).

Although anxiety and ASD co occur in 84% genome-wide association studies (GWAS) show that they do not share a pathway instead the anxiety mainly occurs as a result of the social interaction difficulties and problems caused by the rigid routines (Hallett et al. 2010).

Case of Darren (2007)

Darren was being held in a secure unit for young offenders over 200 miles from his home. He was 15 years old. He had been diagnosed as of average ability with Attention Deficit Hyperactivity Disorder and Conduct Disorders. He had been apprehended for stealing on several occasions, became violent when arrested and had been in the care of Social Services after exclusions from several schools and for absconding when put in Local Authority Care. His mother was a hairdresser and his father worked offshore in the oil industry, an "aloof man." Darren had been difficult to manage from an early age but was a third child in a second marriage and so his mother had built the necessary skills to manage him most of the time at home until recently. She insists he is not hyperactive.

She had learnt to be calm and steady and consistent with him. Any change in his routines could send him into screaming fits that could last all day. He was also highly likely to say inappropriate things about people or to them about their appearance or behaviour and use foul language when reprimanded and throw a temper tantrum.

At 7 years he had been banned from one set of grandparents' home after several incidents. The final straw came when he climbed on the roof of his grandfather's shed and would not come down when told it was dangerous. He told his grandfather where to go and what to do with himself in foul abusive language. His mother felt that the two primary schools that he had been to had learnt to manage Darren fairly well. But this had mainly been to let him do his own thing whenever possible and send for her when he became impossible to cope with. He had also developed learning difficulties possibly as a result of missing learning opportunities and parts of the curriculum. He had been given a Statement of Special Need but this came late in junior school. It was at Secondary school that major problems began to develop. Peers bullied him because of his lack of social skills and immaturity. When he became disruptive in lessons peers encouraged him and often they would set him up to become disruptive. He was easily led. His way of attracting friends was to give them presents of sweets at first. Later he learned to steal to get them presents. Some of the boys told him to do these things and he was guileless and did what they told him. Exclusions followed.

In the secure unit he had come under more dangerous and criminal elements and was being bullied there too. He was becoming more aggressive and frightened.

Vulnerability in ASD

Not only are people with ASD vulnerable to bullying they can become caught up in crime like Darren. This may be inadvertent but because of a special intense interest in e.g., locks or fires; strong dislikes; inappropriate touching; stalking someone they become infatuated with; peeping into windows and all sorts of behaviours that might be tolerated in young children but are seen as bizarre in youths or adults (Howlin, 2006).

Darren for example is guileless and does as his ‘friends’ tell him. This has resulted in his being locked in a secure youth detention centre for behavioural disorders and criminal activity for 18 months. When he comes out he will be 16, with a criminal record and little support or understanding of his problem except by his mother. But now he is too big and disturbed for her to manage hence our consultation.

As can be inferred from this account Darren has Asperger Syndrome and possibly ADD. He also has specific learning difficulties in reading, spelling and handwriting. All the attention was focused on his difficult behaviour and attentional deficits and so he was set upon a ‘career in disruption’ because of a lack of understanding of his Asperger condition. Although progress had been made in the specialist clinical field it had not percolated into his schools and local Care Services.

Darren’s prognosis is poor and it is likely that he will end up in prison despite all his mother’s valiant attempts to help him unless they can access some specialist help. First the family will move to a new area to keep him away from the criminal influences of his ‘friends’. This was the mother’s former home. She is hoping to use the family network to help Darren find a job with an understanding employer. With the Asperger diagnosis she may also be able to find a local network and gain some support for them both.

Preoccupation with children’s difficult behaviour to the exclusion of other diagnoses is not a new problem. Pawley (2007) identified 10 such cases in Year 7 in a London special school for EBD. They all had diagnoses of ADHD and Conduct Disorder but when their literacy difficulties were addressed the problem behaviour diminished by over 50 per cent on the Connor’s Behaviour Rating Scale (2007) in one semester and two specialist lessons per week.

Smith (2002) found that of 20 pupils just referred to a PRU and a Special School, 19 had unidentified dyslexic difficulties and one, a girl had AS. The major preoccupation of the institutions involved was to deal with the challenging behaviours but not to investigate any underlying causes that might help understand and alleviate them.

Walsh and Scullion et al. (2014) found that in 40 cases referred for Conduct Disorders with a primary diagnosis of ADHD, 70 per cent had co morbidity with ASD and/or Dyslexia. Three quarters of the group had language impairment and one third had reading comprehension and reading accuracy deficient scores. The ratio of boys to girls was 3:1.

Gender and Asperger Syndrome

Asperger noted that the condition was much more common in boys than girls. He found it was not usually identifiable before the age of three or even later however autism was most frequently identified around the age of 2 years. Researchers have now identified the conditions within the first few months of life using gaze avoidance and brain scan studies but the average age of diagnosis of AS in the UK is 9 years and many may not be diagnosed until adulthood if at all (Hattersley, 2010). Jenkins (2014) reported a 40-fold increase in diagnosis of AS in the last few years. In the popular press and on radio and television there has also been a corresponding interest in the condition.

The recorded ratio of boys to girls with the condition has varied from 9:1 (Wolff & Barlow, 1979) to 4:1 (Wing, 2008). Over the last few years the number being diagnosed has stabilised after the increase and now is 3.8% per 1000 for boys and 0.8% for girls. The likelihood of a child diagnosed with AS arriving in a class is thus about 1 in 100 individuals (NAS, 2014) but Attwood (2008) claimed 1 in 29 men have AS.

The gender ratio of 4 to 1 raises the question that there could be a failure to identify significant numbers of girls with Asperger just as there has been with dyslexia where the historical ratio of 4:1 (Rutter et al. 1970) has since become 3:2 (Rutter and Caspi et al. 2004; Montgomery, 2008).

Those responsible for referring children for diagnosis are perhaps handicapped by prevailing stereotypes, for example the 'geek' or 'nerd' addicted to computer games, football facts and so on are all associated with boys' behaviours. Whilst it is frequently ignored that girls with total commitment to celebrity, shopping, horses, make-up, or soap operas on TV may be exhibiting their form of Asperger rituals and routines and need further investigation and possible diagnosis and support. Gould et al. (2011) suggested that girls with AS learn to mimic social interactions and communications more easily than boys and learn to act in social settings. Diagnosticians therefore see someone who appears capable and who has reciprocal conversation and uses appropriate affect and gestures. These girls do not appear to fulfill the criteria in the international classification systems and a diagnosis is missed. A checklist is not sufficient to diagnose their needs a case history and wider exploration of actions is needed including their devotion to an interest that is intense and beyond the normal range. If they do attract attention it is likely that their diagnosis will be ODD (Oppositional Defiant Disorder) rather than Asperger Syndrome.

Twice Exceptional Children (2E): Giftedness and AS

Asperger Syndrome has received particular attention from those concerned with research in gifted education when it was realised that a significant number of gifted individuals also displayed Asperger-like symptoms.

It first became apparent that a significant number of autistic people such as Nadia (Selfe, 1977) had isolated 'gifts' usually in music, art, or number calculation. However it can appear in other forms that are not so valued by society such as 'addiction' to the learning of the working of bus or train timetables; naming all the players in the football teams past and present and the goals that were scored in matches. These isolated abilities are typical of 'Savants'.

Some individuals with AS and high abilities have talents in areas involving memory feats and literal activities. This means that school subjects requiring more conventional factual knowledge rather than abstract understanding of ideas can enable them to achieve high scores in examinations. This is until they meet the need for more complex abstractions, perhaps at university level. Even then they can navigate their way through to high achievement by memorising different abstract positions.

Individuals with giftedness and Asperger Syndrome like those with dyslexia and giftedness are regarded as Twice Exceptional or children with Dual Exceptionality (2E). They need support both for giftedness and their special need (Montgomery, 2003, 2014 a, b).

In many cases children with 2E have an additional difficulty or special need in the form of developmental coordination difficulties (DCD) especially in handwriting (Montgomery, 2007). Henderson et al. (2001) found that over 90 per cent of those with Asperger Syndrome had handwriting difficulties. It is these that can radically affect compositional and spelling abilities and access to the curriculum. Teachers are generally very unsympathetic to poor or illegible writing and seem unable to help children overcome them except by rote learning of spellings and demanding neat rewriting (Montgomery, 2008). Technology aids are only a partial solution to this problem.

Providers were becoming confused between what was idiosyncratic gifted behaviour and what was disordered and Niehart (2000) offered guidance on this situation as follows:

Table 2. Similarities and differences between Giftedness and AS

Factors that can be the same	Factors that are different in AS
Verbal fluency, or precocity Early reader, often self-taught	Pedantic seamless speech, lacks appropriateness, understanding is literal
Excellent memory	Mixes fact and personal details
Fascination with letters or numbers	Low tolerance to change, screams if change made
Absorbing interest in a specific topic	may ignore class or school routines completely
Memorises vast quantities of information	Does not understand humour, irony or fables
Annoys peers with endless talk of interest	Lacks insight and affective understanding
Asks awkward questions	Clumsiness in 50-90 per cent
Gives lengthy discourses in answers	Especially may have handwriting difficulties
Hypersensitivity to sensory stimulation	Frequently has stereotypic behaviours or rituals, screams at loud noises refuses to eat this or wear that
High level of skill in one area, average in others	

Typically those with AS may have certain areas of skills such as excellent rote memories, intense interest and knowledge in one or two subjects e.g., astronomy, genealogy, football teams, prehistoric monsters, cars, board games or TV characters in a soap opera. In contrast to the gifted child this interest is to the exclusion of all else, they talk about it endlessly even when the listener is uninterested and shows or even says this. Some less intellectually able individuals with AS may fail to understand the meaning of what they recite. If the interest is in weapons particularly guns then with their lack of social empathy dangerous situations can arise. Although such cases are rare no attempt should be made to support or encourage the interest instead it needs to be replaced by another if at all possible.

Children with AS appear eccentric at school and may be badly bullied and become anxious and afraid. They are unsatisfactory pupils because they follow their own interests regardless of the teacher's instructions and what the rest of the class is doing. There are clues to AS when individuals are involved in playing with a favourite toy or a computer game. If the teacher or parent calls to them by name they do not turn their heads even in a minor social way to signify they have heard. A normal response is to turn and respond or at least move the head and glance towards the adult. Such focused attention can be an attribute in a noisy work setting but dangerous in a hazardous one.

At adolescence many do become aware of their difficulties, but they may then become over-sensitive to criticism and appear very vulnerable and pathetic or very childish. Later it may lead to depression.

Wing (1996) concluded that good self-care, a special ability that can be used in some form of paid employment, and a placid nature are required if the person with Asperger Syndrome is to become socially independent.

"The 3.30 Time Bomb"

Some children with AS go undetected in school but parents report to the National Autistic Society (Hattersley, 2010) that the stresses they have to withstand during the school day build up huge pressures. When they arrive home at 3.30 pm they 'explode' and take out their distress on parents and siblings. They can become unmanageable and inconsolable. Greater cooperation between schools and parents is therefore essential to ameliorate these problems.

Case of Jake, Age 11

Jake was diagnosed with both dyslexia and Asperger Syndrome at 7 years. He was repeating Year Six in mainstream in an International School because the secondary school would not accept a child who needed a Learning Support Assistant and the primary school felt he was not ready to go to the Secondary School.

He had very literal comprehension and did not understand jokes and sarcasm. This made him vulnerable in the playground where he had many altercations. He had difficulties interacting socially and making friends. His behaviour was noticeably immature for his age and he tended to play with younger children. When observed in the classroom it was noticeable that he quickly tended to become over excited. He also found it difficult to modify his behaviour and adapt to different situations.

When asked what he did when the family went on a camping holiday he said, "I went to bed, I ate breakfast. I got dressed."

On another occasion he told a story about how his parents were angry with him after he had cleaned out the goldfish bowl. He had emptied out the fish too and that killed it. He was not upset about this but could not understand why his parents were angry.

Jake liked routine and became very upset if the timetable changed or a new teacher appeared without notice. When he visited the SENCo's room (Special Educational Needs Coordinator) the first thing he did was check that the date had been written on the top right hand side of the board. If it was not he would become very agitated and refuse to begin the lesson until she wrote it there.

Although Jake needed a great deal of support he often refused to take it. Sometimes he refused to cooperate or listen. He would know what he wanted to do which was not always what the teacher wanted him to do. It was then very difficult to persuade him that it was necessary for him to do as he was told.

What we can observe in the goldfish incident is the focus of great attention to the particular and the lack of ability to see the configuration or the bigger picture. This is often why things go wrong and adults fail to understand these 'misdemeanours' and the apparent lack of common sense. Part of the support system needs to include explanations of this focusing ability and it can help promote understanding and remove a lot of anger and frustration the strange acts can engender. Opportunities for employment can be found that will capitalise on such abilities.

This phenomenon of enhanced perceptual focusing can be explained by suggesting 'neurotypicals' have evolved the ability to inhibit raw sensory input in order to form concepts and make decisions more quickly. Creativity could stem from freeing ourselves from these 'top down' interpretations and gaining access to another level of 'bottom up' processing, in the same sort of way as people with AS.

Using a Collaborative Game to Observe and Plan Intervention

"The Egg Race" was selected from Bowers and Wells (1988). There were four different egg characters cut into pieces and each child was given an envelope with a different number of pieces from different eggs. The pupils' task was to assemble puzzle pieces to complete all the eggs correctly.

The rules were:

- No talking or use of sign language.
- No taking pieces from other's puzzles
- You can offer pieces to someone
- You can accept a piece offered by them

Case of Josh, Age 7

Josh (JS) was fairly new to the Year 2 class of 7 year olds. He had been diagnosed with mild AS. He had been assigned some Learning Support Assistant time and with her help he was prepared as far as possible for this different activity that was to be a change from the usual class routine. He was told the activity would be doing puzzles instead of writing.

Josh had a number of eccentric habits that greatly entertained his peers. He used a number of invented words when fussed about a change in activities or answers to questions from the teacher. Jaw clicking, finger clicking and hand flapping would accompany this.

At other times he would perform a whole section of his favourite TV programme Fawlty Towers in the voice and mannerisms of Basil Fawlty. These were very lifelike and funny. He was capable of rerunning a whole programme that he had memorised. Instead of keeping this for playground entertainment he would suddenly start performing as Basil at inconvenient times during lessons.

Telling him to stop had little effect. The teacher had to move in close, talk to him in a quiet a calming manner and show him something interesting to distract him with a new activity or object to switch off the other. (A picture cueing system was recommended to help in this).

The group was told that the puzzle pieces fitted together to make four different 'egg faces' but they did not necessarily have all or some of the pieces for one puzzle. The rest of the rules were then explained as above.

The Observation Session with Josh's Group

Initially, all the pupils just looked at the pieces in front of them and pushed them around without even trying to put them together. They remained totally focused on their own and ignored other peoples' pieces.

Inevitably JS found the situation difficult. He sat rigidly clicking his fingers, repeating loudly and repetitively "Hot king's rock", "Hot king's rock." After the boys had watched JS for a few minutes they began looking across at each other's pieces. These three AR, FL and MN had puzzled frowns and kept looking at the teacher enquiringly as if wanting her to tell them what to do.

Pupil AR noticed that JS had a piece that he needed and reached across the table to take it. He was reminded that he could not take a piece but had to wait until it was offered to him. JS's response was to pull all the pieces close to him and cover them possessively with his arms repeating loudly, "Spemily! Pyloff!"

Eventually FL noticed he had a piece that AR wanted and offered it to him. AR took it but could not work out which piece it fitted with. After several tries with all the pieces he handed it back to FL. FL shook his head and refused to take it back. AR shrugged his shoulders and kept the piece but left it to one side.

MN had watched this exchange and kept looking at his pieces and everyone else's pieces until he realised that he needed to offer FL a piece. This was received with a grin and fitted immediately to correctly form part of an egg. Once AR and MN saw how FL had fitted two pieces together, they looked more carefully at their own pieces and realised that some went together.

Throughout these exchanges JS kept his eyes averted from the others and focused on two of his pieces, intermittently clicking his jaw. The pieces did not fit together but he repeatedly pushed the two together and pulled them apart, while kicking his foot against the chair leg and from time to time shouted his made up words or lines from Basil Fawlty.

By now the other three boys had worked out what they needed to do and were actively looking at each other's pieces and trying to see what they could offer to someone else. The three also used eye contact to communicate their needs. Both FL and AR offered pieces to JS, but he refused to take them despite desperate attempts with facial expressions and head movements to encourage him to accept them. At no time did he make any attempt to offer a piece to the others although they were eyeing them longingly.

AR, MN, and FL swapped pieces amongst themselves until both AR and MN had completed their eggs. FL could not complete his egg because JS had his missing pieces. He also had pieces that JS needed but had refused to take. The group sat watching JS for several minutes but he did not offer any pieces. FL realised that they had reached a stalemate and so he pushed all his pieces over to JS so he could complete two eggs. The puzzle game took 20 minutes to complete.

This is a characteristic response from a child with Asperger Syndrome and adults too. With adults the game is more complex and consists of 'Broken Squares' but the responses are similar. There is a detailed focus on their pieces and a failure to interact or see the bigger picture. It is a revealing game to use in undiagnosed but suspected cases of AS. In a professional development MA class for teachers a newly appointed primary head behaved just as JS had done and became very angry about the task they had been set to do. She left abruptly and colleagues reported that she was having management difficulties with her staff.

What can be done later is to rerun the game and sit alongside the child with AS and quietly step by step pre-programme the behaviours. This involves teaching him or her – 'first look at your pieces – try to fit them together – now look at AR's pieces – does he need one of your pieces? – Now look at MN's pieces - - -'and so on. In a second rerun it can be possible to introduce – 'look at AR's face – is he smiling at you? –Yes? It means he wants that piece – Give it to him'

The game strategy can then be used as a protocol to help him generalise to other situations and develop some social skills e.g., 'Do you remember the game? - 'First I must check what I have got.' – 'Then I must look around to see who or what might help me' - - -.'

Case of Helen, Age 15

Helen was 15 years old when diagnosed with atypical ASD. She is a compliant student keen to do anything required of her. She is always happy in her own company and does not appear to have a close group of friends. She does not participate in conversations unless specifically asked a question.

She seems totally unaware of the comments or actions of those around her but she can be over critical of other students if she feels they are not following the instructions that have been given.

Helen is of below average ability and appears a little aloof when being spoken to. She frequently needs instructions explained several times. She has very good reading and spelling skills but her comprehension is weak. She always requires assistance with compiling and presenting written notes and when asking or answering questions.

She can take a long time thinking and expressing herself, often developing a heavy breathing action as she progresses through the thinking process.

During practical activities Helen is fairly slow and methodical, displaying weak fine and gross motor skills resulting in clumsiness and difficulty working as part of a team, She always tries her best and shows no emotional distress when things are not going according to plan. She is always delighted with the practical items she produces whatever the level of achievement reached.

Her lack of attention to personal hygiene matters and presentation is now an issue.

Helen's is an Asperger profile that we might identify in more girls if we were to look carefully as Gould et al. (2011) suggested. She certainly has Pragmatic Language Disorder and limited awareness and empathy for others' needs.

At this stage she needed a mentor to work with her on the hygiene issues. There are a number of options that can be pursued. The important feature is to establish a set of routines in which a hygiene issue is introduced and dealt with in a step-by-step procedure. It can begin with self-report, a morning diary, or social stories. Each has to be concrete and factual and then when a step is missed discussing what the result would be, how other people might respond and so on. Each aspect has to be applied to Helen's situation and experience e.g., why peers avoid sitting by her or refuse to work with her and so on. Any progress can be reinforced with peer attention and praise plus any tangible rewards that might be appropriate.

Case of Tom, Age 15

Tom was a 15 year-old pupil diagnosed with Asperger Syndrome. He attended regular school and was accelerated in maths, physics, biology and modern foreign languages.

In year 8 he took GCSE's in physics and maths and obtained 'As' in both and passed the extension paper in maths. He was able to follow the 'A' level and scholarship level work with the support of a lecturer from the local university and staff from the school provided enrichment programmes for him so that he gained an 'A star' in biology and an 'A' in French.

Whilst he was capable of advanced work in these academic subjects his social and behavioural skills were a cause of much concern. Staff had referred to his frequent interruptions of lessons. He asked many inappropriate questions not accepting a conversation with a teacher was finished when it was. He had difficulties remaining in his seat and problems working in a group.

At the beginning of Year 9 his teacher (Barber, 1996) decided to develop a special programme to teach him how to take a bus to the nearby city, to begin to prepare him for going to college. On the first visit she paid the fare , They took an agreed route through the city centre and planned what to say if someone asked for directions. The next time, Tom paid the fare and took his tutor on the journey. On the next occasion he went alone whilst she followed the bus in her car and finally he went through the whole process on his own. In his evaluation he wrote:

> 'This was useful as it helped me to gain independence and I learned how to use the bus service. I would like, if it were possible, to do this again, over a longer distance' (p. 21)

Barber went on to develop a behaviour management programme with him to stop him making a fuss, grumbling under his breath, looking as angry as he could and even screaming when asked to do something he did not want to do. When asked why he behaved in this way he said that it was because of his 'urge to learn' and because the teacher often covered work that he already knew.

> Barber's future plans for him were to target skills in shopping, planning a meal and using a telephone.

As can be seen there is an extraordinary range between high abilities and deficits in Tom's case. The deficits are in skill areas that pupils at a much younger age would normally acquire without being directly taught. They are capable of incidental learning of all these necessary social and life skills whereas pupils with AS like Tom may need specific step-by-step instruction in areas of deficit. If his parents had been better supported they might have been able to help him at a much earlier stage. He has been fortunate to meet a well-informed teacher who has clearly helped him.

He is fortunate that he has 'special talents'. These can protect pupils with AS from being excluded or sent to special schools for EBD. Unfortunately there may be only one in ten who have such high ability and special talent. The rest like Darren and Helen have not been so fortunate.

Effective Interventions Used in AS

In relation to whole spectrum of autistic disorders there have been more than 55 different types of interventions proposed according to the National Autistic Society. Some are more effective than others in AS and have been selected for inclusion here.

Behaviour Modification (BM) Now Termed ABA - Applied Behavioural Analysis

Positive reinforcement is widely used to reduce conduct problems in classrooms. It works if applied to specific and small events such as remaining in seat, keeping still and stopping talking. Primary reinforcements such as food and drinks can work better with children with ASD than verbal and social reinforcements when they are young. Teacher approval and praise becomes more significant as they mature. Whilst BM is effective in the initial stages it frequently fails to maintain orderly behaviour in the long term (Montgomery, 1989, 2002) unless the time in between is used to develop new positive behaviours and changes to teaching strategies.

Time out is a commonly used strategy. When behaviour looks likely to disrupt the concentration and learning of other children and the child with AS the 'Time out' routine can be used to establish calm and quiet. There needs to be a time out place, carrel or even a room where the child can go or be taken and allowed to calm. Time out should be for as short a period as possible and the purpose explained – to enable the child to regain control and to become calm again. It can be augmented with a picture cue card as illustrated in the section on the next page.

Modelling. The teacher points out what is desirable behaviour of a peer and positively reinforces successive approximations to it from the AS learner.

Intensive Interaction, This is most often used in autism. It involves close interaction on a one to one basis and begins with mirroring the behaviour of the child and using successive approximations to develop social behaviour and stop unwanted behaviours (Nind and Hewett, 1994).

Social Skills Training (SST)

In a meta-analysis of 79 studies Schneider (1992) found SST moderately effective in increasing social competence in natural settings with socially withdrawn children. But problems arose in the generalisation and transfer to new settings and this is particularly true in AS. They found programmes using modelling and coaching were the most effective.

There are three theories of transfer (Blagg, et al. 1993) implicit in a number of intervention studies.

- The 'Bo Peep' theory: Transfer will take care of itself 'leave them alone and they'll come home'. Their research showed that this was not the case. Learners often failed to deploy or adapt their intellectual and social resources in unfamiliar circumstances.
- The 'Lost sheep' theory: Transfer rarely occurs so most new problems are likely to require additional training.
- The 'Good shepherd' theory: Transfer does occur if it is shepherded, nurtured and mediated by specific teaching and learning activities.

Unfortunately SST studies rarely have control groups and there is a lack of instruments to measure their effectiveness. In AS the social skills are now frequently incorporated into the Social Stories approach outlined below.

Augmented Visual Communication Systems

Symbol systems use the tendency for people with ASD to be visual learners. They provide visual support for communication in the form of objects, photographs, pictures, gestures or line drawing symbols. They are usually paired with the words they represent so that a basic vocabulary can be built for communication purposes in severe autism.

They can be used very effectively in AS to gain and support behaviour control and social interaction. People in conversation use many gestures, signs and facial expressions to support their communications and these can all be taught to help children at home and at school.

Boardmaker Picture Communication System has clear graphics and is in black and white or colour. It includes social words, descriptors, people, verbs and nouns. It has 3000 pictures/symbols and uses simple line drawings of Makaton signs (www.makaton.org) if there is no appropriate picture. Picsyms from Speechmark is similar to Boardmaker but has 1800 picture/symbols.

Case of Sarah, Age 9

Sarah was a 9-year-old pupil with AS in a special school for EBD.
Picture cue cards successfully used:

- Good listening – used as a request to follow instructions or to re-join the class after Time out – picture of head with hand cupping ear
- Good girl – used when she followed the instruction – smiling face with halo
- Good hands – not to hit others – person sitting quietly with hands in lap
- No spitting - a head blowing out a candle
- No screaming – a face with a glum expression and hands over ears and a red line across the picture
- Time out – a chair back to a wall inside a house and blue sky and sun outside - shown when she failed to follow instructions

Football Cue Card System

Red and yellow cue cards can be used by the pupil with AS to warn the teacher that the pressure is becoming too strong and the pupil is suffering distress. Red can be the exit card to go to Time Out and yellow the warning to 'cool it'. Sometimes they cannot find the words to express these feelings.

Dietary Interventions

Allergic responses. Historically various dietary treatments have been effective with some but not others, notably the Feingold diet in which most popular foods with additives are removed. The additives such as tartrazines caused an allergic reaction that provoked ADHD responses in some children.

Casein and gluten. Reichelt (2001) and his colleagues screened 2 million children over a period from 1979-2001 in Norway. They found that the result of a malfunctioning gene was that casein and gluten peptides in milk and flour respectively cannot be properly broken down. This results in abnormally high opioid peptides being found in the urine. The opioid properties lead to the sensory and perceptual disturbances reported by people with ASD and the behavioural disturbances reported by parents, teachers.

Parents have to keep food journals and remove all casein and gluten products from the child's diet. At first they report that the child gets worse as frequently there has been overdosing on milk and flour products. After three days it is typical that a transformation takes place. A non-communicating five year old began speaking in coherent sentences, others began to play constructively and in interaction with siblings and their behaviour came within the normal range.

According to these parents their children still remained on the autistic spectrum but with a less extreme condition much more like a child with AS and able to learn in school and find suitable careers.

These studies were replicated at Sunderland University Autism Research Unit (http://osiris.sunderland.ac.uk/autism)

Dietary Treatment Feedback from NAGC Family

Reports received from parents who have tried the diet with their children are typically inconclusive. For example, one boy in the family was diagnosed with autism and another older gifted sibling was diagnosed with dyslexia. The diet was tried with the autistic boy and the other one participated incidentally because it was simpler for all the family to follow the diet. The result was that the autistic boy's behaviour did calm down and become more manageable but the dyslexic boy became a model pupil and his literacy skills improved as a result. His behaviour had also been extreme and difficult (AS) but the family had hardly noticed because of their concerns with the management of the younger boy.

The diet is always worth trying because if there are no positive effects within a week then it can be discontinued and checked off the 'to try' list.

(NAGC is the National Association for Gifted Children)

Theory of Mind and Social Stories

Baron-Cohen, et al. (1986) proposed that the autistic individual lacked a 'theory of mind'. They showed it was a cognitive deficit that could be observed reliably across a series of studies and resulted in the disorders found in the development of social and communication skills and abilities. They identified 'mind blindness' in autistic individuals as a delay in the development of ability to impute mental states to themselves and others. As a result they find other people's behaviour particularly confusing and worrying.

In simple terms this can be illustrated by their example: *Two people stop and look in a shop window, one points at something in it, the other nods and they go into the shop. Shortly after one of them comes out and looks in the window again and goes back inside the shop. Then they both come out again one with a plastic bag of something.*

The normal onlooker infers that the two people are out shopping, see something one of them might want in the window and go in to buy it. The shop assistant wishes to know exactly where in the window it is and they cannot remember exactly and so one comes out to check and then goes back inside to tell them. We believe the object is bought and put in the plastic back and they leave. If we had no theory of mind about what other people are thinking and doing, all this running in and out of a door in ones and twos would seem very peculiar. A theory of mind gives us a device for understanding social behaviour and ways of interacting and communicating appropriately with others. Without it life would seem very chaotic even frightening and might cause us to withdraw or react in social circumstances in very peculiar ways as though people were objects. It is noticeable and perhaps not surprising that in spoken language individuals with AS seldom use the words 'know, believe, think, pretend' as many teachers will be aware. It becomes particularly obvious in the early years play and later in English lessons in role-play and imaginative writing. The mental state of attribution is necessary if in our talk with others we are to respect the conversational rules of pragmatics - if it is to be appropriate and relevant to the social context.

> In a room, Sally places a marble in a basket in front of her (location A). Anne in the same room has a box in front of her (location B). Sally exits the room and while she is absent Anne transfers the marble from the basket to her box.
>
> The question is - where will Sally look for her marble when she comes back into the room?

The answer is of course in A because she believes that it is still where she put it. 86% of children with Down's syndrome and 85% of normal children passed this test whereas only 20% of autistic children did so. This was despite the autistic children being older mentally and chronologically than the others. All were required to have a verbal mental age of 4 years to understand the narrative but only had to respond by pointing.

80% of the autistic children chose location B where the marble actually was. This result was stable over many replications by different researchers in subsequent years (Frith, 1991).

Even the 20% who passed the 'belief' test appear only to do so at the first order level, that is, Sally thinks X. They were found to have impairment and fail at the second order belief or attribution level - Mary thinks that John thinks X whilst this is well within a normal six year olds' understanding (Baron-Cohen et al. 1986).

The 'mind blindness' aspect of autism may enhance some talents because autistic individuals do not see the configurations that 'neurotypicals' do. Baron Cohen (2008) went on to develop the theory of a cognitive deficit to include a deficit in social empathy and an above average ability in systematising (imposing order and structure) to account for the triad of impairments.

Social Stories: Gray, 1990, 2003

These are short stories developed by Gray in the US that describe social situations in terms of relevant social cues and effective responses. They are often colourful and visually illustrated to clarify the meaning of communication, conversations and social situations.

The stories give the children the reason why things happen and, direct them in understanding how they should react in a particular situation, what they should say, what they should do and then explains why. The purpose is to make social rules and conventions explicit to the child with AS whereas the rest of children infer these principles and procedures implicitly. The stories are very short and give the child a protocol of four types of sentence. These are:

- Descriptive - explain where and what
- Perspective - explain feelings and behaviour of others
- Directive - state what the child is expected to do
- Control - strategies the child can use to remember

In using the protocol Gray advised using one directive and / or control statement to every two to five descriptive / prescriptive statements. The method works in the following way:

- Sometimes my friend Tom tells me to 'chill' (descriptive)
- This means I am getting loud and bossy (descriptive)
- Tom does not want to sit with me when I am loud and bossy (perspective)
- I will lower my voice when Tom tells me to chill (directive)
- When Tom tells me to 'chill' I can imagine putting my voice on ice (control) (Gray, 1990, p. 223)

Gray's original comic strips and stories are now enhanced by DVDs www.graycenter.org

Teenage Needs – A Group Problem

A typical problem identified by a group of Year 11 secondary school boys with Asperger Syndrome was that they were desperate to learn how to 'chat up' a girl they would like to have a date with. They just did not know how to go about it.

Their special teacher/mentor with the help of colleagues in English and drama designed some role-play situations that began with a simple meeting and greetings taking place between two people. The teachers modelled the behaviour, video clips were shown of others' meetings and the boys practiced the sequence and were coached. They learned to make eye contact, smile a little, lift the eyebrows in recognition and offer a standard greeting. They were encouraged to practice this in the corridors at school with people they knew.

They progressed from these scenes to learning to make a short set of interactive statements that might encourage a potential partner to meet them again.

They were taught the conversational routines of looking and listening and turn taking, how to stand and not confront, not to touch or stand too close. All of this was reinforced in role-play and a group of girls joined in to act as 'buddies' and give feedback and help.

The boys all found this approach helpful. Their teachers felt that their social approaches had improved but the use of the conversational protocols was somewhat rigid in 11 out of the 12. They hoped that with experience these would loosen up a little and be used more flexibly. As can be imagined this would be extremely difficult for most of the boys.

Education for AS Some General Principles

There is no known treatment that has any effect on the basic impairments but the handicaps can be diminished by appropriate management and education that involves:

- Regular organised routine
- Careful communication with the pupil and parents
- Modification of repetitive speech and motor habits
- A highly structured visual learning environment
- Use of visual prompts and written instructions
- Sensitive use of behaviour modification
- Development and extension of the special interests
- Learning broken down into short concrete logical steps

- Teachers with good social and calming skills
- A tolerant supportive school environment.

These techniques are freely available to all teachers in regular classrooms.

In AS there are usually few problems in gaining a range of GCSEs that require factual knowledge but it is the social difficulties that cause great concern and that mean they will need some form of care or support in adult life. Their extreme need for absolute regularity and routine in which the slightest change requires them to be very carefully prepared is also of major concern for it means that the simplest interaction in a shop or in employment can be unpredictable and disturbing to them and cause an overreaction.

Mainstream Inclusive Learning - The AS Friendly School

Curriculum

- Visual timetables with pictures and symbols to support the routines.
- Diaries and computer schedules when pupils can read, to show the routines and especially any changes that are due during the day
- A timer to show the passing of time and to regulate the completion of work, teach what 'finished' means.
- Plan for independent work and give the pupil folders 'Work to complete' and 'Work completed' to aid organisation and prediction.
- 'Visual organisers' to help structure subject contents and procedures
- Give directions or limited choices as free choice can induce anxiety
- Arrange that class activities as far as possible can be taught in small steps or that a worksheet, computer programme or LSA (Learning Support Assistant) can act as a step organiser
- Avoid the use of abstract ideas or tasks such as 'imagine', 'invent' unless specific strategies are taught to handle these
- Give help in ensuring that skills learnt in one context can be generalised to new situations
- Introduce new ideas or procedures gradually, always checking for understanding
- Each aspect of the 'hidden curriculum' needs to be taught
- Avoid using metaphors, fables and figures of speech in the teaching process e.g., 'My feet are killing me', 'It is raining cats and dogs'. If they are essential or appear in books they need to be explained.

Social

- Teach the specific rules of turn-taking, social distance and gambits for opening and maintaining a conversation

- Learn calming techniques and strategies such as agreed gestures, signs and calming voice and statements
- Address the child individually by name at all times to focus attention before any communication
- Make clear with a firm 'No' and gesture or sign what is unacceptable
- Give enhanced supervision during practical and physical activity
- Arrange a 'Buddy' system and 'circle of friends' to support and protect the pupil
- Avoid sarcasm, the hidden meaning will not be understood
- Protect from teasing and bullying. The school must have a policy on bullying
- Do not take apparently rude or aggressive behaviour personally

Environment

- Ensure that the learning environment is quiet and orderly, too much noise can create anxiety or lead to disruptive outbursts
- Make sure the classroom is not cramped or overcrowded
- Use sound damping carpet and wall coverings where possible.
- Have a study carrel to use as a retreat, or a quiet corner with beanbags for younger children and a 'Time out' room
- Ensure the pupil has a personal workspace and a place to keep belongings
- Organise regular breaks for relaxation in a play area for young children or perhaps using 'Brain Gym' for older pupils.
- Avoid white walls, stripy clothes, whiteboards, and fluorescent or bright lights. Black mats in front of doors may be perceived as black holes; murky painting water in the sink may appear to cut off the hands and provoke screaming.
- Avoid moving the furniture about unless the pupil has been prepared.

School-home and staff liaison

- Ensure there is good home/school liaison as parents have key information and experience to share and can support the school
- Ensure there is inservice development on AS for all staff including administration staff, cleaners and dinner helpers etc. so that they can understand and avoid confrontation and asocial comments

Such a long list is challenging but not every item is called for in every situation or raised in every case.

Case of Peter, Aged 18

Peter was in Year 13 in a small Catholic comprehensive school. He was from a disadvantaged city background. Neither parent had ever been in work or had any form of advanced education.

He has mild AS showing clumsiness, poor social skills and literal comprehension. He finds it difficult to adapt to any new situation or change in routines but it does not provoke strong behavioural outbursts.

At GCSE (Year 10) he achieved 9 A stars, 2 A's and a B. In Year 12 he gained an A in Maths. His maths teacher/mentor determined he should apply for university although many others who had taught him were against the plan. They said he would not cope in an open learning environment and one so full of new and different experiences and social demands.

Peter refused to go on the school's week study tour of a number of universities. He was however finally persuaded to go on a residential visit to one university. The whole sequence of buying tickets, journey planning accommodation and transport to and from the railhead were gone over in detail and executed with his tutor. He had never been away from home and his parents were against the university project. However he was impressed with the place and the facilities.

With intensive training he managed to fill in the UCAS form finding the business of writing, acquiring stamps, cheques, photographs, photocopies and envelopes extremely frustrating. His first trip and interview went well but he was not offered a place. However it boosted his confidence to have succeeded in making the trip and finding he could master it all.

At his second and third choice universities he was offered a provisional place depending on gaining good grades – AA BB, which in due course he did. He accepted a place at the campus university that his mentor thought more suited to his needs.

His mentor arranged with Student Services to offer him support as soon as he arrived and that his new maths tutor should also be involved to engage with his needs.

Counteracting Curriculum Difficulties

Pupils like Josh have difficulty with many aspects of the curriculum especially in English and History. These subjects put particular cognitive demands on them because of the everyday tasks that teachers set such as 'Imagine', 'What did X intend to do?' and especially 'Why' questions.

Where curriculum subjects are confined to the literal and factual then pupils with AS will be able to flourish and even gain A* results at GCSE. Particular difficulties may ensue in some of the practical tasks in Science and Design because of the inherent coordination difficulties. More problems can result from subjects requiring a lot of handwriting. Word processing will be easier and should be encouraged with the provision of laptops where there are handwriting difficulties.

In examinations those with writing difficulties should be awarded extra time and this can be applied for from the examining authority as for those with dyslexia needing extra writing time. In the most severe cases a scribe may be necessary and appropriate training and practice given.

Imagine

When the children are asked to imagine they are in novel situations or in a different time or place the pupil with AS will find this task impossible and will not know where to begin. S/he will not have a concept of what it is that you could possibly want. In this situation some tasks can be modelled in a literal way. For example:

Imagine that you get up one morning and find you are only 25 cm tall. Describe what happens to you during a school day.

This is a typical task that might be set in primary school. After a 'brain storming' session most pupils will find a way to start on their stories. However younger children and the pupil with AS may need to make a manikin and walk it round the room to see the concrete difficulties encountered. When teamed up with a 'buddy' each can tell the other what is happening at different stages on the journey. With a little encouragement situations in the home can be modelled such as having breakfast or getting up and washing.

The key events can be recorded like a scientific experiment as they happen to the toy. Toys and finger puppets can be extremely useful to model what otherwise would be imaginary activities.

Imaginative poetry is also difficult but so much of the best of it begins with very close observation of something a flower, a pylon, a drop of water. This close observation even using a lens can lead to detailed observations that can be worked into poems. English teachers usually have a basket of these strategies on hand to support learners, for example. *The Full English* Blake (2006) and www.teachit.co.uk

How do you think you would feel if -?

This is another problematic area. In a similar fashion to the toy scenes, children engaged in role-play can 'see' important scenes played out that enable them to write about an imaginary event. Video clips, pictures and playlets depicting important subjects will help because they provide the visual support the child needs to understand the world.

Debriefing is a particularly important part of teaching and learning because the pupil will need attention directed to the key points and the deeper meaning of many events and actions that would otherwise pass them by.

The structure of the Social Stories provided by Gray in the section above can provide the framework and direction for showing the pupil with AS how things appear to other people and how they might be feeling. As the pupils grow older they can use such structures as a scaffold for themselves and learn to direct their attention and behaviour in a strategic manner.

Why?

Because pupils with AS lack a 'theory of mind' they find it hard to move from the literal to hypothesise about ideas and events. For example:

- Why did Hitler invade Poland? "He hated the Poles."
- Why did Juliet die in the play Romeo and Juliet? "Because she took poison."
- Why was money invented? "So we can buy things."

Scaffolds

These can be particularly helpful in guiding pupils with AS in all their composing and writing tasks. The scaffolds can be presented in the form of a series of pictures or cartoons, or as short sentences that guide them through typical tasks. The simplest one that we use with young children in story writing is to get them to understand that stories have a beginning, middle and end. We might give them the scaffold in a series of boxes (visual organisers) in which they can write notes preparatory to writing the story or narrative.

Taking this a stage further we can read them some beginnings from well-known stories so that they can identify the type of beginning and how the scene is set. Then the class can practice making beginnings e. g.

- Atmosphere - It was cold and dark, the fog just began to drift towards - - -
- Place - The house was small, built of red brick and was in a corner of the square- -
- Time - It was very early, he knew this because - -
- People - Jack was tall and well built - -
- Period - The harbour was full of sailing ships preparing for the battle - - -

Thinking Actively in a Social Context (Wallace 2000). The TASC wheel is a widely used resource scaffolding for creative problem solving. The 8 steps are: Explore knowledge: Identify the problem: Generate ideas: Decide on one: Implement: Evaluate: Communicate: What have I learnt?

An experimental intervention in the English curriculum

Harbinson and Atkinson (2009) identified 12 pupils in their secondary school with AS statements. They asked both the pupils and their teachers what difficulties were encountered in English lessons. They then gave the pupils an imaginative writing task to establish a baseline before their interventions and analysed previous work.

Their analysis of examples from a Key Stage 3 (14 years) exam illustrated the problems pupils with AS would face even though they had an option to describe a real event e.g., –

> Write a story describing a frightening experience.
> This may be based on a real or imaginary experience. It may be serious or amusing.
> In your story you should give information and describe - -

They observed that even if the pupils could make a response the mark scheme would discriminate against them. They would be unable to attain the higher levels in the marking scheme such as:

- presents reflections on feelings
- shows development of a personal style
- engages the reader's interest (p. 12)

Equally difficult were the inferential reading skills required in questions such as –

> What do you learn about Darcy from reading lines 21-69 in the passage?

Here, at the higher levels the mark scheme required –

- analysis of aptly selected references (connections difficult to make in AS requiring generalisation from parts to wholes)
- present convincing insights (insight into own and others' actions and ideas is absent)
- offer perceptive understanding (mission impossible!) (p. 13)

Even though the task allowed for literal interpretation the pupil with AS may still not know how or where to begin. The word 'imagine' may have aversive connotations from past difficult experiences. Some learners with AS even regard imaginative stories as 'telling lies'. Others may have learnt to rely entirely upon an LSA to guide them through the task. Now in a large inclusive classroom, support may have to be shared or even be absent.

The research programme ran over 16 weeks cut into two 8 week blocks, section one of whole class teaching and section two in which the pupils with AS were withdrawn in groups of 4 for one hour a week for the intervention. Then there was a post-test.

The programme involved two types of input on:

1. A specially designed creative writing framework - Who? When? Where? What? Why? with visual cues and prompts.
2. An inferential reading skills scaffold in three sections
   i) What did he say? What did he mean?
   ii) What did he do? What does this show?
   iii) How would you feel?

The result was that in the first 8 weeks despite the scaffolds being taught to and used by the whole class including the pupils with AS, no progress was made.

In the second 8 week period the intervention in groups allowed more interaction, and informal talk about the tasks and where stories came from and so on. This was a little more successful.

The 3 English teachers involved in the study identified the following range of problems in the pupils with AS:

- Engaging in talking and listening
- Inferential reading
- Decoding figurative language
- Empathy skills
- Starting new tasks that expect imagination
- Analysing a character in a piece of fiction
- Knowing how to deal with a mistake (p. 14)

These pupils needed the preparation to begin in primary school and be reinforced across the curriculum for it to be internalised, the 'Good Shepherd' approach. The suitability of the 'training' scaffolds also needs to be questioned. Many schools embrace the policy of inclusion but do not action it or train their teachers appropriately.

Donna Williams (1996) a high functioning adult with autism explained:

> "I am diagnosed as having autism ..... If you ask me what the word means, I would tell you that, for me, it is about having trouble with connections... this also causes trouble with tolerance and trouble with control..." (p. vii)

* making connections - problems in attending to parts and not perceiving the whole; lacking sensory integration - seeing but not hearing or able to listen at the same time, accumulation of information but lacking any organisation of it and needing triggers for recall.
* tolerance - problems in sensory and emotional hypersensitivity making input unpredictable and overwhelming, sometimes there is fear of own voice or other people's.
* control - problems of compulsions, obsessions and acute anxiety, so may rock to calm self down.

Conclusion

Improving self-management skills will assist in integrating pupils with AS into regular classrooms. It must start from the earliest moment at home and continue throughout education. Improving communication skills reduces the need for deviant communications. These interventions need to be cumulative, developed in appropriate contexts and transfer of the training needs to be ensured through modelling, coaching and extended practice.

As can be seen in most of the cases outlined in this chapter the interventions are occurring too late and need instead to be part of a lifelong learning plan. As knowledge advances we can hope that this will be shared and parents and teachers can develop the necessary skills to help children with AS find their place in society. Improving and extending parent partnerships with schools is essential to this process.

The Case of Sonia, Age 11

Sonia is 11 years old and has a diagnosis of mild AS. After a series of upsets and being bullied in primary school her parents have decided that she would fare better in a small private secondary school with a good reputation for helping children with special needs.

Sonia is a pretty child with blonde hair and blue eyes. She looks sweet but has a habit of making very unacceptable remarks about people. Her new teacher understands the condition but the Learning Support Assistants did not. When Sonia announced that one was too fat and the other had a big bum they were shocked and hurt. Their anger and disapprobation only made her worse and it was difficult to stem their complaints and her behaviour.

Sonia was unaware she had done anything wrong and began hand flapping and marching round the room muttering. When an LSA tried to stop her Sonia began screaming.

The reader is invited to think through what should have been done in Sonia's case and how the school can help her.

References

ASPEN (Asperger Syndrome Educational Network) http://www.asperger.org accessed March 3rd 2014.

Asperger, H. (1979) 'Problems with infantile autism' *Communication* 13 45-52.

Attwood, T. (2008) *The Complete Guide to Asperger's Syndrome* London: Jessica Kingsley.

Barber, C. (1996) 'The integration of a very able pupil with Asperger Syndrome into mainstream school' *British Journal of Special Education* 23 (1) 19-24.

Baron-Cohen, S., Leslie, A.M. and Frith, U. (1986) 'Mechanical, behavioural and intentional understanding of picture stories in autistic children' *British Journal of Developmental Psychology* 4 123-25.

Baron-Cohen, S. (2008) 'Theories of the autistic mind' *The Psychologist* 21 (2) 112-16.

Bishop, D.V.M. (1989) 'Autism, Asperger Syndrome and Semantic-pragmatic disorder. Where are our boundaries?' *British Journal of Disorders of Communication* 24 107-21.

Blagg, N.R., Ballinger, M.P. and Lewis, R.E. (1993) *Development of Transferable Skills in Learners*: *Research Series* Sheffield: The UK Government Employment Department.

Blake, J. (2006) *The Full English: An A to Z of English Teaching Activities* Sheffield: National Association for the Teaching of English www.nate.org.uk.

Boardmaker Picture Communication Symbols (1981-92) Mayer-Johnson Co. P. O. Box 1579 Solana Beach CA 92075 USA.

Bowers, S. and Wells, L. (1988) *Ways and Means; A Problems Solving Approach,* Kingston upon Thames: The Friends Workshop Publication.

Connors, C.K. (2007) Connor's Comprehensive Behaviour Rating Scale, London: Pearson, Psychological Corporation.

Dehaney, R. (2000) 'Literacy hour and the literal thinker: The inclusion of children with semantic-pragmatic language difficulties in the literacy hour' *Support for Learning* 15 (1) 36-40.

DfEE (1998) *The National Literacy Strategy Framework for Teaching* London: Department for Education and Employment.

DfEE (2001) *The Code of Practice Revised* London: Department for Education and Employment.

Frith, U. (ed.) (1991) *Autism and Asperger Syndrome* Cambridge: Cambridge University Press.

Gabis, L., Raz, R. & Kesner-Baruch, Y (2010) 'Paternal age in autism spectrum disorders and ADHD' *Paediatric Neurology* 43 (4) 300-302.

Gould, J. & Ashton Smith, J. (2011) Good Autism Practice www.autism.org.uk accessed 3rd March 2014.

Gray, C. (1990) *The Social Stories Book* Arlington TX: Future Horizons.

Gray, C. (2003) *My Social Stories Book* London: Jessica Kingsley.

Hallett, V., Ronald, A., Rijsdijk, F. & Happe, F. (2010) 'Association of autistic-like internalising traits during childhood' *American Journal of Psychiatry* 167 (7) 809-17.

Happe, V., Ronald,A. & Plomin, R. (2006) 'Time to give up on a single explanation for autism' *Nature Neuroscience* 9 (10) 1218-20.

Harbinson, H. & Alexander, J. (2009) 'Asperger syndrome and the English curriculum: Addressing the challenges' *Support for Learning* 24 (1) 11-18.

Hattersley, C. (2010) 'Autism factfile' *Special* 24-6.

Henderson, S.E. and Green, D. 2001 'Handwriting problems in children with Asperger Syndrome' *Handwriting Today* 2 65-71

Howlin, P., Iverson, M. & Gilbert, C. (2004) 'Teaching and learning approaches for children with Asperger's Syndrome - Literacy Implications and applications *Teaching Exceptional Children* 36 (4) Council for Exceptional Children.

Howlin, P. (2006) Crime vulnerability in ASD International Conference on ASD, Cardiff.

Jenkins, J. (2014) 'Out of the ordinary' BBC, Radio 4 11.30-12.00 3rd March.

Kanner, L. (1943) 'Autistic disturbances of affective contact' *The Nervous Child* 2 217-50.

MAKATON www.makaton.org

Montgomery, D. (1989) *Managing Behaviour Problems* Sevenoaks: Hodder and Stoughton.

Montgomery, D. (2002) *Helping Teachers Improve through Classroom Observation* London: David Fulton.

Montgomery, D. (2003) *Gifted and Talented Children with SEN: Double Exceptionality* London: David Fulton.

Montgomery, D. (2007) *Spelling, Handwriting and Dyslexia* London: Routledge

Montgomery, D. (2008) 'Cohort analysis of writing in Year 7 following 2, 4 and 7 years of the National Literacy Strategy' *Support for Learning* 23 (1) 3-11.

Montgomery, D. (2014) a *Autistic Spectrum Disorder; Study Guide M10* Maldon: Learning Difficulties Research Project www.ldrp.org.uk

Montgomery, D. (2014) b *Dual and Multiple Exceptionality: Study Guide M16* Maldon: Learning Difficulties Research Project www.ldrp.org.uk

National Autistic Society (NAS) (1997) *Approaches to Autism (3rd edition)* London: National Autistic Society www.autism.org.uk accessed 9th March 2014.

Niehart, M. (2000) 'Gifted children with Asperger's Syndrome' *Gifted Child Quarterly* 44, 4 222-30.

Nind, M. & Hewett, D. (1994) *Access to Communication: Developing the Basics of Communication with People with Severe Learning Difficulties Through Intensive Interaction* London: David Fulton.

Reichelt, C. (2001) 'Biochemical basis for autism' The Food Programme, Radio 4 14th January 2001.

Rommelse, N.N., Franke, B. Geurts, H.M. et al. (2010) ' Shared heritability of attention deficit/hyperactivity disorder and autism spectrum disorder' *European Child and Adolescent Psychiatry* 19 (3) 281-95.

Ronald, A. (2014) 'The times they are a-changin' *The Psychologist* 27 (3) 144-66.

Rutter M. L., Tizard, J. and Whitmore, N. (1970) *Education, Health and Behaviour* London: Longman.

Rutter, M. L., Caspi, A., Fergusson, D., Horwood, L.J., Goodman, R., Maughan, B., Moffatt, T.B., Meltzer, H.C. & Carroll, J. (2004) 'Sex differences in developmental reading disability' *Journal of the American Medical Association* 291 9, 16, 2007-2012.

Rutter, M. (2005) 'Genetic influences and autism' 425-52 In F. R. Volkmar, R. Paul, A. Kline & D. Cohen (eds) *Handbook of Autism and Pervasive Developmental Disorders 3rd edition* Hoboken, NJ: John Wiley and Sons.

Schneider, B.H. (1992) 'Didactic methods for enhancing children's peer relations: A quantitative review.' *Clinical Psychology Review* 12 363-82.

Selfe, L. (1977) *Nadia: A Case of Extraordinary Drawing Ability in an Autistic Child* London: Academic Press.

Speechmark Ltd www.speechmark.com

Wallace, B. (2000) *Teaching the Very Able Child: Developing a Policy and Adapting Strategies* London: David Fulton.

Walsh, I.P., Scullion, M., Burns, A., MacEvilly, D. and Brosnan, G. (2014) 'Identifying demographic and language profiles of children with a diagnosis of ADHD' *Emotional and Behavioural Difficulties* 19 (1) 42-59.

Williams, D. (1996) *An Inside Out Approach* London: Jessica Kingsley.

Wing, L. (2008) Asperger Syndrome: A clinical account www.mugsy.org/wing2.htm (Accessed 24/03/2008).

Wing, L. (1996) *The Autistic Spectrum: A Guide for Parents and Professionals* London: Constable & Co.

Wing, L.(1981) 'Asperger Syndrome: A clinical account' *Journal of Psychological Medicine Reprint:* Autistic Society.

Wing, L. and Gould, I. (1979) 'Severe impairments of social interaction and associated abnormalities in children' *Journal of Autism and Childhood Schizophrenia* 9 11-29.

Wolff, S. and Barlow, A. (1979) 'Schizoid personality in childhood: a comparative study of schizoid, autistic and normal children' *Journal of Child Psychology and Psychiatry* 20 29-46.

In: Asperger Syndrome
Editor: Michael F. Shaughnessy

ISBN: 978-1-63463-810-4

Chapter 11

Group Social Skills Intervention for Adolescents with Asperger Syndrome or High-Functioning Autism Spectrum Disorder: Curriculum, Process, and Outcomes

***Tammy D. Barry*[*1], *James K. Goodlad*[1], *Theodore S. Tomeny*[2] *and Elizabeth C. Fair*[1]**
[1] The University of Southern Mississippi, MS, US
[2] The University of Alabama, AL, US

Abstract

Given that social impairment is a key feature of autism spectrum disorder (ASD)—including individuals diagnosed with Asperger Syndrome—social skills training remains paramount. This chapter describes the curriculum for an outpatient clinic-based social skills group intervention for high-functioning adolescents with Asperger Syndrome or ASD and presents the results of analyses examining the process and outcomes associated with the implementation of the group. After completing an initial assessment, six adolescent males (aged 12 to 17 years) with an estimated IQ within the Average range or above (i.e., high functioning) and a previous diagnosis of Asperger Syndrome/ASD were admitted into the group intervention. In addition, five typically-developing peers from local high schools attended the group as social models. Each session included five general components: a warm-up activity to promote group interaction; an instructional component to teach new skills; snack time to promote unstructured practice of new skills; guided role-play and active practice of new skills; a review of skills discussed/ conclusion, and assignment of homework to facilitate practice of skills outside of the group. Parents were provided a review of each session, including the skills covered and assigned homework for the adolescents. Each week's session focused on a new social

[*] Tammy D. Barry, Ph.D., The University of Southern Mississippi, Department of Psychology, 118 College Drive, #5025, Hattiesburg, MS 39406-5025; Email: tammy.barry@usm.edu.

skill, including getting to know others and starting a conversation, turn-taking in conversation and activities, self-monitoring of appropriate and inappropriate comments, perspective-taking, nonverbal communication and intentions behind comments, understanding emotions in self and others, and social problem solving. In addition to measuring cognitive functioning and ASD symptomatology before group participation, behavioral/emotional functioning and social skills of the ASD group members were assessed before the group and at the last meeting using parent-report measures. Group leaders completed the Therapeutic Alliance Scale for Children (TASC-R). A descriptive analysis of pre- to post-intervention changes indicated modest improvement on global behavioral measures following participation in the 8-week group intervention, particularly for externalizing behaviors. Unexepectedly, internalizing symptoms (particularly depression and somatization) tended to increase from pre- to post-test. Furthermore, analyses with the TASC-R demonstrated a marginally significant negative correlation between group leader alliance and autism symptom severity, shedding some light on how therapeutic alliance may have an impact when professionals are working with adolescents with Asperger Syndrome or high-functioning ASD.

Keywords: Autism spectrum disorder, Asperger Syndrome, social skills group

Introduction

Autism spectrum disorder (ASD) is a developmental disorder characterized by deficits in social and communication skills and the presence of restrictive or repetitive behaviors (DSM-5; American Psychiatric Association, 2013). Asperger Syndrome was previously considered a separate diagnosis from autism—both of which were under the umbrella of pervasvive developmental disorders (DSM-IV-TR; American Psychiatric Association, 2000). However, with the implementation of DSM-5, indviduals who would have previously been diagnosed with Asperger Syndrome in DSM-IV are now described as part of the autism spectrum. In general, indivdiuals with Asperger syndome function similarly to indivdiauls with high-functioning ASD. Throughout this chapter, reference to individuals with ASD would include also individuals diagnosed with Asperger Syndrome.

Given that social deficits are a key feature of ASD—including for those with high-functioning ASD or Asperger Syndrome—therapies aimed at improving social skills are often necessary to help individuals with ASD learn how to engage in appropriate social interactions. Because of the significant role of social interactions during adolescence, therapy services addressing the social skills of adolescents with ASD are particularly important. Adolescents with ASD who lack an understanding of social situations or appropriate ways to interact with others may have more difficulties forming friendships and may be at risk for loneliness or for developing depressive or anxious symptoms (Bauminger, Shulman, & Agam, 2003; Strang et al., 2012). In fact, adolescents with ASD are at an increased risk to report having higher levels of depression, lower-quality friendships, more loneliness, and increased peer rejection and bullying (Bauminger & Kasari, 2000; Bauminger et al., 2003; Chamberlain, Kasari, & Rotheram-Fuller, 2007; Humphrey & Symes, 2010; Locke, Ishijima, Kasari, & London, 2010). Therefore, interventions aimed to improve social skill development among those with ASD remains paramount.

Cognitive and behavioral techniques have consistently been shown to improve outcomes across a number of different problem areas. More recently, these techniques have been applied to help children, adolescents, and adults with ASD learn social skills. In particular, techniques that include the establishment of "social rules" through didactic discussion and Socratic questioning (e.g., Laugeson & Park, 2014), modeling and role-playing (e.g., Nuernberger, Ringdahl, Vargo, Crumpecker, & Gunnarsson, 2013) of both appropriate and inappropriate skills, and the inclusion of ecologically valid homework assignments (e.g., Barry et al., 2003) have demonstrated success in achieving social skill acquisition. Based on the success of these previous programs and to minimize the possibility of negative long-term outcomes, we implemented a group social skills program to target social deficits in adolescents with ASD.

The program targeted seven social skills that have been found to be especially difficult for adolescents with ASD. For example, research has shown that individuals with ASD have difficulties initiating conversations and beginning friendships (Knott, Dunlop, & Mackay, 2006; Lord & Magill-Evans, 1995; Müller, Schuler, & Yates, 2008). Lord & Magill-Evans (1995) reported that children and adolescents with ASD tended to initiate less than typically-developing peers and also were less likely to coordinate introductory behaviors with eye contact. In addition, even when these individuals did initiate peer interactions, their initiations were less successful. Because of these difficulties, initiating conversations was the first major target of our intervention. Individuals with ASD have also shown difficulties associating with peers and understanding how to maintain socially-appropriate conversations once a social interaction has already been started (Knott et al., 2006; Luteijn et al., 2000; Müller et al., 2008). Therefore, developing skills with respect to turn-taking and self-monitoring of appropriate and inappropriate comments were the second and third targets of our group.

The ability to take the perspective of others and understand someone else's point-of-view is critical for any social interaction. It has been well established that individuals with ASD tend to struggle with understanding others' mental states and perspectives (e.g., Baron-Cohen, Leslie, & Frith, 1985), so the fourth target of our skills group was increasing perspective-taking abilities. Likewise, understanding nonverbal communication and nuances of social interactions can be very difficult for individuals with ASD (Lutejin et al., 2000). Thus, the fifth target of the group was addressing nonverbal communication and intentionality in social interactions. Research also suggests that individuals with ASD have difficulties understanding complex social emotions, something that is necessary for social interactions to be effective. For example, a study conducted by Capps, Yirmiya, & Sigman (1992) found that individuals with ASD had more difficulties explaining social emotions such as pride and embarrassment. Specifically, participants with ASD needed more time and prompting to discuss these emotions, had more scripted responses, and had more limited understanding than typically-developing peers. Because of these deficits, the sixth target addressed emotion understanding. Finally, the aforementioned deficits often lead individuals with ASD to struggle with social problem solving and generating appropriate responses to difficult social situations. For example, a study conducted by Bauminger et al. (2003) found that individuals with ASD had more difficulties generating ideas for how a lonely child could join a group. Additionally, individuals with ASD self-reported difficulties determining how to behave in various social situations (Knott et al., 2006). Therefore, social problem-solving was the seventh target of the group.

In summary, adolescents with ASD display social deficits in a wide variety of areas. Our social skills group was created to help address common deficits identified by researchers and to improve social functioning in adolescents with ASD using empirically-supported intervention strategies. This intervention utilized group-based cognitive-behavioral techniques in an outpatient setting via didactic social skills lessons and in-session, supervised practice of skills with five high-functioning adolescents with ASD. The current study examined behavioral, emotional, and social outcomes as well as the nature of the therapeutic alliance between participants and clinicians.

Method

Participants

Group participants were five Caucasian males aged 12 to 17 years (M = 14 years) with a diagnosis of ASD. All participants were communicative, able to participate in a verbal educational environment, and were considered to have high-functioning ASD/Asperger Syndrome. Participants ranged from 100 to 127 (M = 111.8, SD = 10.52) on the Gilliam Asperger's Disorder Scale (GADS; Gilliam, 2001) and from 24 to 42 (M = 33.6, SD = 7.16) on the High-functioning Autism Spectrum Symptom Questionnaire (ASSQ; Ehlers, Gillberg, & Wing, 1999). One participant discontinued group participation after two meetings; therefore, post-test outcome data is only available on four participants.

Cognitive functioning of all participants was assessed using the Wechsler Abbreviated Scales of Intelligence (WASI; The Psychological Corporation, 1999) to ensure appropriateness of fit in the group prior to participation. Each participant earned an estimated Full Scale IQ score > 85 (M = 96.25, SD = 10.34). Therefore, all group participants were considered to have high-functioning ASD.

Five typically-developing peers from local high schools also attended the group. These teens participated fully in the group discussions, role-plays, and activities as social models. They also were assigned and completed the social homework provided to the participants with ASD. Typically-developing peers received community service credit for their participation in the group.

Sequence and Content of Sessions

With the exception of Session 1, which spends a considerable amount of group time orienting adolescents to the program, each session followed the same basic structure (outlined below in greater detail), including a warm-up activity, review of the previous session's content and homework discussion, didactic instruction of the new topic with group discussion, snack time, active practice, and closing. Additionally, parents were debriefed on each week's session content and homework assignment, provided a letter written by the group leaders containing a brief description of the content, and were encouraged to review skills included on the homework worksheet with their adolescent and help facilitate the completion of homework.

Each 2-hour group session was led by two Master's level clinicians. Adolescents received approximately 1.5 hours of direct skills training and active structured practice guided by the clinicians. The remaining 30 minutes allowed opportunities for the spontaneous practice of skills (and clinical observation/assessment by the clinicians). Although sessions were highly structured and session content was predetermined, clinicians were allowed flexibility in their implementation of the program and in the degree of emphasis placed on the various components of each session's didactic lessons to meet the overall strengths and weaknesses of the group members. Clinicians were encouraged to pause and address specific questions about the content of each meeting and not remain too rigid in the overall structure of the group. However, enough structure needed to be imposed each week to ensure that each topic was covered appropriately with enough time for both formal and informal practice and behavioral rehearsal. It is also important to note that sessions and session content often built upon the previous week's content. Specifically, basic skills like appropriately beginning and ending conversations or using appropriate body language were mastered first before addressing higher-order skills such as social problem-solving, appropriately communicating one's needs, and understanding the subtle social cues of others. An additional benefit to structuring sessions this way was that prerequisite skills continued to be practiced each week in different social contexts (i.e., as part of higher-order skill practice) to increase generalization of the skill.

Warm-up Activity

Most warm-up activities consisted of social games that were designed to be fun, while also encouraging group participation and increasing cohesion. Warm-up activities were typically related directly to the session's didactic content. As such, these activities often allowed leaders to actively assess the strengths and weaknesses of the group in that area and to anticipate any difficulties in delivering the content. Each session's warm-up activity is described in more detail below.

Social Homework Review

Each week following the active practice portion of group time, the previous session's content was briefly reviewed with the group, and members were encouraged to share their homework. Adolescents were given worksheets created by the group leaders outlining each session and the accompanying assignment to serve as reminders of the material covered in each session and what they needed to practice at home and in the community. Parents were also encouraged to review each adolescent's homework and help him or her complete the worksheet as needed. Group time was first spent reviewing the work of individuals who successfully completed homework assignments. Time was then spent problem-solving with adolescents who were unable to complete the assignment. In all, there was some variability in homework completion. Common reasons cited by the group members for not completing the social homework included that they lost the assignment, did not understand the assignment, or did not have an opportunity to complete the assignment, among other cited barriers. However, again, any problems brought forward were discussed so that these barriers would not prevent the completion of future social homework assignments.

Didactic Instruction and Group Discussion

Each session's content was first presented through a didactic and lecture format. Group leaders took turns presenting content and writing key points, phrases, or rules on the board so that group members had an opportunity to learn both visually and verbally. Following the presentation of rules, leaders used open-ended questions about the content to spur discussion typically focused on the reasons why a particular rule is important or identifying good examples of skills in action. Group leaders continued to moderate this discussion by calling on members who participated appropriately (e.g., by raising their hand) and shaping answers of the group so that they aligned with the social rules. For off-topic or inappropriate responses, group leaders often posed open-ended questions to the group as a whole (e.g., "What might be the problem with that?") rather than directly challenging the adolescent to avoid embarrassing the adolescent or providing unnecessary attention to distracting behavior.

Snack Time

Snack provided a much-needed reprieve for group members during the two-hour session, as most sessions were conducted in the afternoon following a full day at school. Dietary restrictions were considered and a variety of snacks were provided. A secondary purpose of snack was to provide an informal time for group members to practice skills among each other and for group leaders to appropriately model skills one-on-one with group members. Group leaders also made clinical observations about the group members' implementation of skills in a less structured setting, and this clinical assessment data could be used to further hone skills (e.g., during active practice). Typically-developing peers also ate snacks alongside the adolescents with ASD, providing further opportunities for modeling and natural feedback.

Active Practice

The active practice portion of each session provided the opportunity for adolescents to take the skills they were taught and apply them in simulations of practical situations created by the group leaders to promote generalization of skills beyond the lecture. Each session's active component was specific to the session's content to account for the group's development of skills over time. Often, group leaders predetermined the order of practice or the pairs and groups in which adolescents practiced to ensure that each adolescent with Asperger Syndrome or high-functioning ASD had an appropriate number of peer models. Group leaders carefully monitored the active practice, provided coaching during each adolescent's practice of the skill, and guided the group in providing appropriate feedback to the adolescent.

Note on the Inclusion of Peer Models

One unique aspect of this program is the inclusion of typically-developing "peer models" (i.e., typically-developing adolescents who actively participated in the group but who did not have a diagnosis of ASD). Although group leaders spent considerable time teaching skills through lecture, modeling skills among themselves, and role-playing skills with the group, the inclusion of peer models in each of the group activities provided invaluable same-age behavioral examples of age- and developmentally-appropriate social skills. Occasionally, peer models also served as behavioral coaches during group by directly helping adolescents with ASD learn and practice skills. Peer models were carefully screened prior to the group and participated only after they agreed to attend and participate in each group and complete the weekly social homework.

Group Sessions

Session 1. Session 1 began with group leaders introducing themselves and allowing each member of the group to introduce himself or herself by first name only. A warm-up activity requiring each adolescent to say their own name and introduce each group member who went before him or her was meant to be a fun, interactive way to begin building relationships among members, and it allowed for a baseline assessment of basic social skills by the group leaders. Following the completion of this activity, group leaders oriented adolescents to the basic structure of group. Leaders provided adolescents with information about the format of group, the topics that were to be presented over the next eight sessions, and the purpose of "social homework" assignments between sessions. It was also important for group leaders to review basic group rules. These rules were not pre-determiend; however, group leaders explained behavioral expectations during group and encouraged members to generate appropriate rules as a group. Many of the adolescents with ASD were able to generate several suitable rules (e.g., raising one's hand to speak, keeping hands to self, being respectful). Leaders also explained the group's point system in which adolescents could earn up to five points per session by attending, following rules, and actively participating throughout the meeting. Participants were able to bank their points to be used during the wrap-up session at the end of the eight weeks to "buy" a prize.

The goal of the first session's didactic component was to ensure that adolescents learn appropriate ways to introduce themselves and trade information. Leaders wrote down rules for greeting others (e.g., make eye contact, smile, say "hello," introduce yourself, ask the other person for his/her name, wait for a response). The first session's active practice occurred during snack time and consisted of providing each group member with a list of peers in the group, predetermined by group leaders, with whom to trade information. Each list contained both peer models and other group members with an ASD. The group was also provided with ideas for questions to ask peers (e.g., favorite hobbies, sports, or subject in school) and leaders periodically checked in with each adolescent to provide coaching as needed. At the end of the activity, homework was assigned: meeting someone new and trading information with them to bring back to the group.

Session 2. The main goal of Session 2 was to increase each adolescent's understanding and ability to take turns in conversation. After rules were briefly reviewed, adolescents were split into subgroups with an equal number of participants with an ASD and typically-developing peers for a warm-up activity. Group leaders modeled appropriate introductions and then each subgroup took turns introducing their members to the larger group and, within each subgroup, members took turns introducing each other (i.e., Member 1 introduces Member 2, who introduces Member 3, and so on). Additionally, participants were encouraged to include information learned from the previous week. A major focus of the activity was on turn-taking and this was highlighted for group members.

After reviewing homework, Session 2 focused on turn-taking both in conversations and activities. Key points in the didactic portion of the session included allowing others to take turns in conversations, how to offer others a chance to participate in groups, and how you do not always have to be the first to participate or speak while in a group. After snack, during which group leaders monitored the use of turn-taking skills informally, active practice was a game show-style activity in which adolescents took turns being the "decision maker" for their team. However, they were also encouraged to give the whole team a chance to discuss the best answer among each other before an answer was provided by their decision maker.

Session 3. Session 3 focused on self-monitoring and evaluating what kinds of comments are appropriate and inappropriate around different groups of people (e.g., family, friends, acquaintances). This session's warm-up activity was a "Have You Ever?" game in which group leaders created note cards with a "have you ever...?" question on it (e.g., "Have you ever been on a sports team?" "Have you ever been to the beach?"). Group members then took turns asking the group questions using the note cards to determine the most popular and rare activities completed by the group members. The didactic lesson about monitoring appropriate versus inappropriate comments covered four key areas, including making positive self-statements without boasting and responding to compliments, appropriately communicating when something is unfair, accepting and getting along with people who act or think differently than you, and receiving criticism appropriately. For active practice, leaders demonstrated role plays in which group members were provided hypothetical situations meant to promote the use of new skills by acting out both positive and negative examples of handling the situation. Meanwhile, the rest of the group was asked to identify if and how statements could have been improved by allowing time to "stop and think" before speaking. For homework, adolescents were encouraged to use "stop and think" skills to self-monitor, manage, and decrease their use of inappropriate comments.

Session 4. Session 4 addressed an aspect of perspective taking by exploring others' points-of-view and the higher-order skill of understanding intentions underlying comments and nonverbal cues beyond their literal meaning. The session emphasized the need to take the perspective of the other person to better understand their possible intentions. The warm-up activity consisted of a group problem-solving game based on the story of the Blind Men and the Elephant. In this story, a group of blind men come across an elephant but do not know what they have encountered given that they cannot see it. Each man touches a part of the elephant (e.g., tusk); yet, because they individually only encounter a small part of the elephant, they do not realize that they have found an elephant. However, if they consider all of the information provided by each man in the group as a collective, they are able to conclude that they have found an elephant. Group members were provided with single clues and they were encouraged to work together to solve the riddle by taking each other's perspective.

The didactic section about intentions behind comments and nonverbal cues of others stressed several rules, including that one action or statement can have different meanings, it is important to "stop and ask" before jumping to conclusions, and that we cannot always tell what others are thinking or feeling just by what they say (i.e., circumstances are important to consider). Group discussion was generated by presenting members with note cards depicting social situations, and adolescents were asked to comment on how characters felt, what they might be thinking, and how each adolescent may have a different point-of-view of the situation. Active practice involved a game of charades during which group members acted out different situations and others attempted to guess their intentions, emotions, or thoughts. Homework involved observing and recording thoughts and emotions of yourself and how these may change after considering another person's perspective.

Session 5. This session highlighted the importance of accurately identifying emotions in oneself and others. In place of a warm-up activity, the group was divided into members with and without ASD (although it was not labeled that way for the group members). Each group engaged in an overview with one of the group leaders. Members with ASD were reminded of group rules, the importance of earning points, and were shown their current point totals as an incentive for continued participation. Members without ASD (i.e., peer models) were debriefed separately by a leader about ways to continue to encourage group members with an ASD and problem-solve any difficult or uncomfortable situations that may have occurred.

The didactic for identifying emotions in others included several points that tied in directly with the previous session (e.g., it is sometimes difficult to tell how others are feeling, consider the context, integrate information from facial expressions, body language, words, and tone of voice). Identifying emotions in oneself focused on the cognitive-behavioral model related to feelings, thoughts, and behaviors. Group members learned "chill out" skills that included relaxation and thought awareness techniques. For active practice, group leaders modeled and led progressive muscle relaxation, and group members took turns acting out emotions nonverbally for the rest of the group to identify. For homework, members were asked to complete an emotions diary and practice their "chill out" skills.

Session 6. Session 6 began with a review of how difficult it can be to understand the emotions of others, and group members were encouraged to discuss their successes or difficulties and the implications of being aware of others' emotions when taking their perspectives. Adolescents were encouraged (but not required) to share an entry in their emotions diary and discuss their use of "chill out" strategies. Session 6 was the first of two sessions to deal with social problem-solving. Social problems (problems that require coping skills as well as an ability to make choices that lead to favorable outcomes for self and others) were defined and adolescents were taught the PICC model (i.e., Problem Identification, Choices, and Consequences), which was adapted from the Coping Power manual (designed to improve social problem solving among aggressive or behaviorally disordered children; Lochman, Wells, & Lenhart, 2008). Participants were encouraged to "PICC apart" the problem. Leaders helped the group generate examples of social problems and ways to apply the PICC model. The PICC "Maze Game" was introduced for active practice in which social problems were identified and possible choices listed. Adolescents then went to corresponding rooms within the clinic for each choice, and they generated consequences based on the choice. The activity was intended to be a concrete example of how different choices can lead to different consequences. For homework the group was provided with a "PICC Apart Your Problems" worksheet to record their use of the skill before the next session.

Session 7. Social problem solving continued as the topic of Session 7. Group members participated in a hypothetical "Trouble at Sea" exercise. This activity required them to negotiate among themselves which items to throw overboard and which items to keep if they were on a sinking ship. Group members were encouraged to evaluate consequences and use perspective taking skills to understand differences in opinion and ideas about which items to keep. The didactic lesson focused on the PICC model with an emphasis on "slow down" and "stop and think" instead of acting on one's first choice.

The majority of the session entailed active practice as the group was divided into different teams to create "commercials" for use of the PICC model. First, social problems were independently generated by each team. Teams then wrote brief scripts for three possible solutions to their social problem. After scripts were finalized, leaders helped each team film their commercial of them acting out each of their three solutions. For social homework, worksheets were provided to help members apply and record PICC model use with specific problems (e.g., being teased or bullied, peer pressure, perceived unfairness). An additional homework assignment was to bring a personal item to the next and final session for show-and-tell.

Session 8. Session 8 began with a presentation of show-and-tell items by each member while group leaders promoted the use of appropriate conversational skills learned in earlier sessions (e.g., sharing the conversation, asking questions of others). The didactic lesson in Session 8 was replaced by a discussion of a social skills review workbook provided to all group members. The workbook provided a brief overview of all of the skills taught in the previous seven sessions, including social rules and social scripts. It also had pages for group members to write about their favorite part of group and their contributions to group. Finally, there were pages for group members to write messages in each other's workbooks (similar to a school yearbook).

Group members were encouraged to review the workbook on their own and discuss the contents with caregivers to increase generalization and continued use of learned skills. A graduation party was awarded to the group for their participation and a pizza party was provided. While enjoying their pizza, group members watched their PICC model commercials and provided the other team feedback. A brief graduation ceremony was then held. Group members with an ASD were awarded a certificate of completion and a selected prize based on the number of points they had earned during the eight sessions. Peer models were awarded a certificate of their service and a gift card to a local retailer. Parents were debriefed and thanked for their participation. Treatment summaries and referral information (if necessary) were provided.

Measures

Wechsler Abbreviated Scale of Intelligence (WASI; The Psychological Corporation, 1999). This standardized, individually-administered, abbreviated intelligence test was designed for individuals aged 6 to 89 years old to obtain an estimate of intellectual functioning. Adolsecents with ASD were administered the two-subtest version of the WASI, including nonverbal reasoning (Matrix Reasoning) and verbal reasoning (Vocabulary). These two subtests yield a norm-referenced WASI IQ score (similar to a Full Scale IQ), with a mean of 100 and a standard deviation of 15. The test has been shown to be reliable (split-half, r = .81, and test-retest, r = .83 to .95). The WASI correlates significantly with the WISC-III FSIQ (r = ,81), showing good construct validity (The Psychological Corporation, 1999). The WASI IQ is appropriate for use as an estimated IQ score (The Psychological Corporation, 1999).

High-Functioning Autism Spectrum Symptom Questionnaire (ASSQ; Ehlers et al., 1999). The 27-item ASSQ asks parents to rate symptoms associated with high-functioning autism and Asperger Syndrome on a scale including *no*, *somewhat*, and *yes*. Scores are summed for a total score, with evidence for cut-offs consistent with a diagnosis of high-functioning autism. The ASSQ demonstrates good inter-rater and test-retest reliability and shows good concurrent and divergent validity in support of its criterion validity (Ehlers, 1999).

Gilliam Asperger's Disorder Scale (GADS; Gilliam, 2001). The GADS is a measure for individuals aged 3 to 22 years which is designed to help identify children/adolescents who may have Asperger Syndrome. Parents complete 32 items consisting of objective, frequency-based ratings. Evidence for both reliabilty and validity support the measure's stated purpose of screening for possible Asperger Syndrome (Gilliam, 2001).

Social Skills Rating System (SSRS; Gresham & Elliot, 1990). The Social Skills scale of the SSRS was used as a broad measure of social functioning (Gresham & Elliott, 1990). The Social Skills scale consists of subscales measuring prosocial skills including cooperation, assertion, self-control, and responsibility. Parents were asked to rate the frequency of their child's behavior on a 3-point Likert scale on 38 items. The SSRS has been shown to demonstrate good reliability and validity (Gresham & Elliott, 1990).

Behavioral Assessment System for Children-2nd edition-Parent Rating Scale (BASC-2-PRS; Reynolds & Kamphaus, 2004). The BASC-2 is a multi-dimensional assessment system that measures both adaptive and problem behaviors of children. Parents rate items on a 4-point scale ranging from *Never* to *Almost Always*. The clinical scales that loaded on the eternalizing, internalizing, and behavioral sumptom composites were of interest. Reynolds and Kamphaus (2004) reported good internal consistency, with alpha coefficients for the composites ranging from .85 to .93 and alpha coefficients for the subscales ranging from .77 to .87. The BASC-2 also has demonstrated good reliability (Reynolds & Kamphaus, 2004).

Therapeutic Alliance Scale for Children-Revised (TASC-R; Ormhaug, Jensen, Wentzel-Larsen, & Shirk, 2014; Shirk, 2003). The TASC-R consists of 12 items that measure emotional aspects and degree of task collaboration present in the therapeutic process. Items are rated on a 4-point scale from *not at all* to *very much*. For the current project, the two group leaders compled the TASC-R in relation to their emotional response and perception of collaboration to each of the group members, following completion of the final group session. The TASC-R has demonstrated good reliability in previous studies (Ormhaug et al., 2014).

Measurement Procedures

IQ was determined through administration of the Weschler Abbreviated Scales of Intelligence (WASI) prior to inclusion in the group. Pre-group data were collected of ASD symptoms via the Gilliam Asperger's Disorder Scale (GADS), amd the High-functioning Autism Spectrum Symptom Questionnaire (ASSQ) completed by parents. Pre-post social skills data were collected via the Social Skills Rating System (SSRS) and pre-post broadband functioning via the Behavioral Assessment System for Children-2nd edition-Parent Rating Scale (BASC-2-PRS). Group leaders completed the Therapeutic Alliance Scale for Children-Revised (TASC-R) at post-group.

Results and Discussion

As discussed in the participant section, group averages—as well as indivdiual data—indicated that the group members were each high-functioning (in terms of intellectual functioning via the WASI) and that their pervasiveness and severity of symptomatology were consistent with high-functioning ASD or Asperger Syndrome (as measured by the GADS and ASSQ).

Mean *T*-scores on the clinical scales of the BASC-2-PRS at pre- and post-intervention are presented in Figure 1. Normatively, *T*-scores have a mean of 50 and a standard deviation of 10. Any *T*-score above 70 is considered clinically significant, and *T*-scores from 60 to 69 are considered at-risk. Compared to normative expectations, as a group, the adolescents with ASD were elevated on hyperactivity, depression, atypicality, withdrawal, and attention problems—resulting in an elevated behavioral symptoms index (composite score).

When examining pre- to post-test changes descriptively, some externalizing behaviors (e.g., hyperactivity, aggression) as well as atypicality tended toward improvement. Other externalizing domains (e.g., conduct problems, attention problems) appeared to be relatively stable. Although there appeared to be a slight decrease in anxiety from pre- to post-test, withdrawal appeared stable—and, contrary to expectation, levels of depression and somatization (i.e., bodily complaints) showed an upward trend from pre- to post-test.

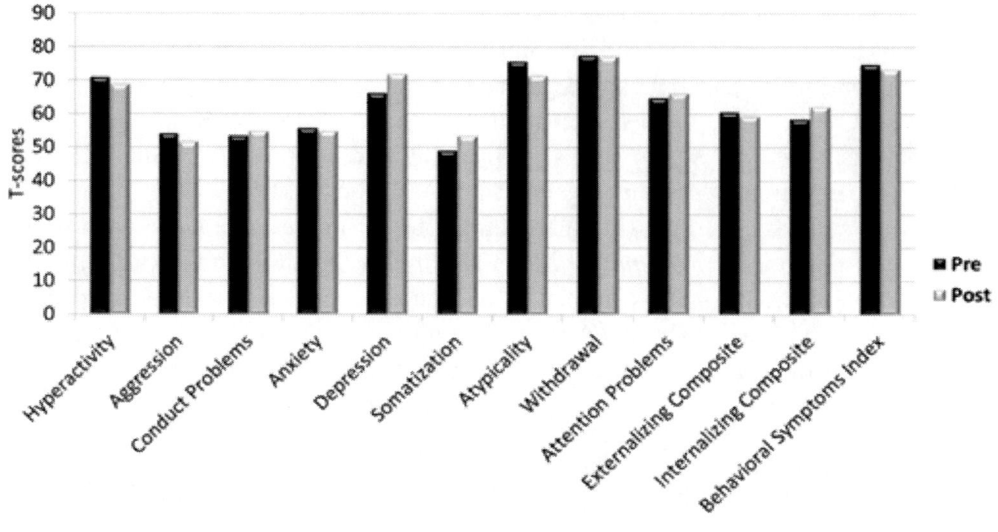

Figure 1. BASC-2 Scales Pre and Post T-scores.

Mean raw scores on the domains of the SSRS at pre- and post-intervention are presented in Figure 2. Descriptively, adolescents with ASD appeared to be more cooperative and to exhibit better self-control following the group intervention. However, responsibility appeared to remain stable, whereas assertiveness skills showed a downward trend.

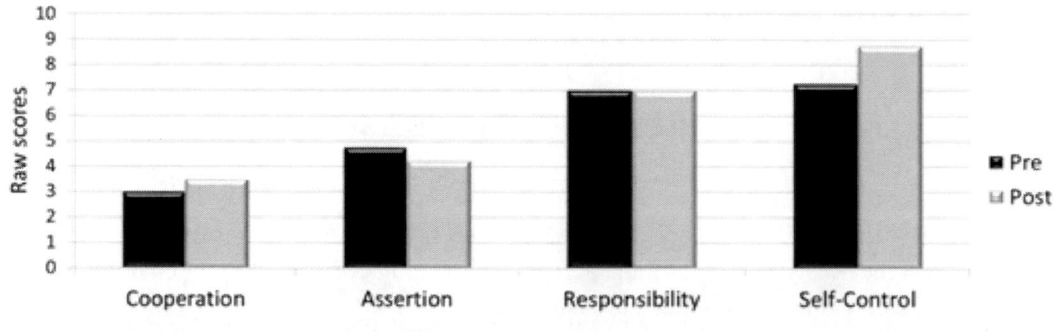

Figure 2. SSRS Pre and Post Raw Scores.

Finally, a strong negative correlation, although only a statistical trend, was observed between group leader ratings on the TASC-R and ASSQ scores ($r = -.92$, $p = .08$). Thus, there was a tendency for group leaders to report a poorer alliance as autism symptom severity was higher. None of the correlations between therapeutic alliance and behavioral, emotional, or social outcomes at post-test were significant, and all such correlations demonstrated relatively weak effect sizes.

The small number of participants in the group (i.e., only four participants with full data available) precluded an examination of pre- and post-test improvement using inferential statistics. However, this descriptive analysis of pre- to post-test scores across measured domains was promising in some aspects. Specifically, although modest, our results showed post-treatment improvements across several parent-report domains of behavioral, emotional, and social functioning after the eight-week intervention. It appears that externalizing behaviors and social skills were the most likely targets for improvement following the social skills intervention. With more extended treatment and additional follow-up, effects may have been stronger. Contrary to expectation, depressive symptoms and somatic/bodily complaints demonstrated slight increases (descriptively). In future implementations of a social skills intervention, such as the one described here, specific additional components to the intervention should be used to address these types of internalizing symptoms—particularly given that depression and loneliness are common problems among adolescents with high-functioning ASD or Asperger Syndrome (e.g., Bauminger et al., 2003). This particular group intervention did aim to target some internalizing symptoms but primarily focused on anxiety (e.g., progressive muscle relaxation, "chilling out"). Depressive symptoms were only targeted more indirectly (e.g., through increasing social skills that may lead to more friendships and less loneliness). Perhaps if more time were allowed before the assessment of depressive symptoms so that the adolescents could implement the social skills learned and make the subsequent gains from those skills, better results would have been realized.

The large negative correlation between group leaders' alliance with group members and group members' ASD symptom severity suggests that clinicians should be cognizant of their own viewpoints and biases when working with children and adolescents with high-fucntioning ASD or Asperger Syndrome. That is, even with treatment gains in other behavioral, emotional, or social areas, alliances were less strong when ASD symptoms were most evident. Knowledge of such potential biases can keep group leaders in check when working with this clinical population.

Overall, this study adds to the evidence that outpatient clinic-based social skills interventions can be beneficial for children and adolescents with ASD. Considerable work remains to determine the best methods for improving social skills interventions for children and adolescents with high-functioning ASD and Asperger Syndrome overall. For example, future research should examine possible variables related to attrition (e.g., diagnostic comorbidity, poor client-clinician alliance, poor parent-clinician alliance) and active components of the social skills treatment package that may strengthen interventions. It is also important to determine if social skills taught and improved upon in the clinic setting generalize to other settings. Although the results from this current investigation are somewhat mixed and conclusions are limited by the number of participants, feedback from all involved—clinicians, adolescents with ASD, typically-developing peers, and parents—indicated that it was a feasible format that was fun, engaging, and informative.

References

American Psychiatric Association. (2013). Diagnostic and statistical manual of mental health disorders: Fifth edition (DSM-5). Arlington, VA: Author.

American Psychiatric Association. (2000). Diagnostic and Statistical Manual of Mental Disorders, Fourth edition, Text Revision (DSM-IV-TR). Washington, DC: Author.

Barry, T. D., Klinger, L. G., Lee, J. M., Palardy, N., Gilmore, T., & Bodin, S. D. (2003). Examining the effectiveness of an outpatient clinic-based social skills group for high-functioning children with autism. *Journal of Autism and Developmental Disorders*, 33, 685-701.

Baron-Cohen, S., Leslie, A. M., & Frith, U. (1985). Does the autistic child have a 'theory of mind'? *Cognition,* 21, 37-46.

Bauminger, N., & Kasari, C. (2000). Loneliness and friendship in high-functioning children with autism. *Child Development,* 71, 447-456.

Bauminger, N., Shulman, C., & Agam, G. (2003). Peer interaction and loneliness in high-functioning children with autism. *Journal of Autism and Developmental Disorders*, 33, 489-507.

Capps, L., Yirmiya, N., & Sigman, M. (1992). Understanding of simple and complex emotions in non-retarded children with autism. *Journal of Child Psychology and Psychiatry,* 33, 1169-1182.

Chamberlain, B., Kasari, C., & Rotheram-Fuller, E. (2007). Involvement or isolation? The social networks of children with autism in regular classrooms. *Journal of Autism and Developmental Disorders,* 37, 230-242.

Ehlers, S., Gillberg, C., & Wing, L. (1999). A screening questionnaire for Asperger syndrome and other high-functioning autism spectrum disorders in school age children. *Journal of Autism and Developmental Disorders,* 29, 129-141.

Gilliam, J. E. (2001). Gilliam Asperger's Disorder Scale. Austin, TX: PRO-ED.

Gresham, F. M. & Elliott, S. N. (1990). Social Skills Rating System. Circle Pines, MN: American Guidance Service

Humphrey, N., & Symes, W. (2010). Perceptions of social support and experience of bullying among pupils with autistic spectrum disorders in mainstream secondary schools. *European Journal of Special Needs Education,* 25, 77–91.

Knott, F., Dunlop, A. W., & Mackay, T. (2006). Living with ASD How do children and their parents assess their difficulties with social interaction and understanding?. *Autism,* 10, 609-617.

Laugeson, E. A., & Park, M. N. (2014). Using a CBT approach to teach social skills to adolescents with autism spectrum disorder and other social challenges: The PEERS® method. *Journal of Rational-Emotive & Cognitive-Behavior Therapy,* 32, 84-97.

Lochman, J.E., Wells, K., & Lenhart, L. (2008). Coping Power: Child Group Facilitator's Guide. New York: *Oxford University Press.*

Locke, J., Ishijima, E. H., Kasari, C., & London, N. (2010). Loneliness, friendship quality and the social networks of adolescents with high-functioning autism in an inclusive school setting. *Journal of Research in Special Educational Needs*, 10, 74-81.

Lord, C., & Magill-Evans, J. (1995). Peer interactions of autistic children and adolescents. *Development and Psychopathology*, 7, 611-626.

Luteijn, E. F., Serra, M. M., Jackson, S. S., Steenhuis, M. P., Althaus, M. M., Volkmar, F. F., & Minderaa, R. R. (2000). How unspecified are disorders of children with a pervasive developmental disorder not otherwise specified? A study of social problems in children with PDD-NOS and ADHD. *European Child & Adolescent Psychiatry,* 9, 168-179.

Müller, E., Schuler, A., & Yates, G. B. (2008). Social challenges and supports from the perspective of individuals with Asperger syndrome and other autism spectrum disabilities. *Autism,* 12, 173-190.

Nuernberger, J. E., Ringdahl, J. E., Vargo, K. K., Crumpecker, A. C., & Gunnarsson, K. F. (2013). Using a behavioral skills training package to teach conversation skills to young adults with autism spectrum disorders. *Research in Autism Spectrum Disorders,* 7, 411-417.

Ormhaug, S. M., Jensen, T. K., Wentzel-Larsen, T., & Shirk, S. R. (2014). The therapeutic alliance in treatment of traumatized youths: Relation to outcome in a randomized clinical trial. *Journal of Consulting and Clinical Psychology,* 82, 52-64.

Reynolds, C.R., & Kamphaus, R.W. (2004). Behavioral assessment system for children (BASC-2). Circle Pines, MN: *AGS Publishing.*

Shirk, S. R. (2003, November). Relationship processes in youth CBT: Measuring alliance and collaboration. Paper presented at meeting of Association for the Advancement of Behavior Therapy, Boston, MA.

Strang, J. F., Kenworthy, L., Daniolos, P., Case, L., Wills, M. C., Martin, A., & Wallace, G. L. (2012). Depression and anxiety symptoms in children and adolescents with autism spectrum disorders without intellectual disability. *Research in Autism Spectrum Disorders,* 6, 406-412.

The Psychological Corporation (1999). Wechsler Abbreviated Scales of Intelligence. New York: Harcourt Brace and Company.

Brief Author Bios

Tammy D. Barry, PhD, is a clinical child psychologist and an Associate Professor at The University of Southern Mississippi, Department of Psychology. She is the Director of Clinical Training for USM's doctoral program in clinical psychology. Dr. Barry's research focuses on contextual and biologically-based correlates of child psychopathology, including attention-deficit/hyperactivity disorder (ADHD), autism spectrum disorder (ASD), and aggressive behavior.

James K. Goodlad, MA, is a clinical child graduate student at The University of Southern Mississippi and predoctoral psychology intern at The University of Alabama-Birmingham's Civitan-Sparks Clinics. His research interests focus primarily on environmental contributors to ADHD and other disruptive behavior disorders. He has recently accepted a post-doctoral position at Civitan-Sparks Clinics to focus on the assessment of developmental delays (including Autism Spectrum Disorder) and disruptive behavior disorders as well as the treatment of social skills deficits in high-functioning adolescents with autism.

Theodore S. Tomeny, PhD, is a clinical child psychologist and Assistant Professor at The University of Alabama, Department of Psychology. His research focuses on the functioning of families of individuals with Autism Spectrum Disorder (ASD) and related disorders and explores factors associated with quality of life of those with ASD, treatment adherence, and generalizability of treatment outcomes. Psychopathology in children and adolescents, both with and without developmental disabilities, is another area of general interest of Dr. Tomeny's research lab.

Elizabeth C. Fair is a graduate student in the Clinical Psychology doctoral program at The University of Southern Mississippi. Her concentration area is clinical child psychology, and her research interests focus on the relation among neuropsychological functioning and expressed behaviors in children with autism spectrum disorder (ASD).

In: Asperger Syndrome
Editor: Michael F. Shaughnessy

ISBN: 978-1-63463-810-4

Chapter 12

A Parent and Teacher's Perspective on Asperger's

Kimberlee Rutan McCafferty[*]
University of Maryland, College Park, MD, US

Abstract

This paper will provide an overview of the issues that a parent and teachers encounter when working with or parenting a child with Asperger's. This paper will review the diagnostic process, the IEP process, sensory issues and coping with challenging behaviors, and the teaching of social skills. In addition, the Individual Transition Plan, and post-secondary training issues will be examined. Finally, independent living, either in a sheltered workshop, college or independent living will be explored.

Keywords: Asperger's, education, daily living skills, transition

Introduction

I am a former educator who has had students with Aspergers in my classroom, and mother to an eleven-year-old with severe autism and a seven-year-old with high-functioning autism. My younger son Zachary developed typically until he was twenty months old, then had a significant period of regression after he suffered back-to-back illnesses. Within a matter of weeks he had lost six to twelve months of development in the areas of fine and gross motor ability, receptive and expressive language, cognition, and social and emotional development. He lost all but a few of his words, and began to suffer severe gastrointestinal issues. His entire demeanor changed from a generally happy child to one who seemed perpetually cranky, enmeshed almost entirely in his own world.

[*] Corresponding author: Kimberlee Rutan McCafferty. E-mail: berleekim@hotmail.com.

Since Zachary's older brother has severe autism, my husband and I already knew how to address the situation. We immediately called Early Intervention for an evaluation, and put Zach on a six month waiting list to see a developmental pediatrician for what we knew would eventually be an autism diagnosis. We used more of a Floortime approach with our younger son (the methodology created by Dr. Stanley Greenspan which advocates "meeting children where they are and builds upon their strengths and abilities through interacting and creating a warm relationship" (The Greenspan Floortime Approach, 2014) working with him twenty to thirty hours per week.

Zach seemed to have more intestinal issues after eating foods with gluten in them, so we removed gluten and casein (dairy) from his diet, and within a week or two began to see results. Over the course of a few months Zach's skin cleared up, his chronic diarrhea lessoned, and he regained some of his vocabulary. The light seemed to return to his eyes.

The Diagnostic Process

After what seemed to be an interminable wait, we eventually got in to see a developmental pediatrician, who at twenty-six months gave Zachary the diagnosis of autism. The term "high-functioning autism" was not in as much use in 2008 as it is presently, and there were no further delineations in his label. By the time we entered the developmental pediatrician's office it was clear to me and my husband that Zachary would not be following his older brother to the severe end of the autism spectrum. Zach had significantly increased his vocabulary by that time, and most of his pleasant personality had returned.

The behaviors that placed him on the spectrum were primarily his restricted and repetitive interests (as in his obsession with Thomas trains). He also had a somewhat limited interest in social interaction with those around him, particularly with individuals with whom he was not familiar. Some of Zach's physical movements were also clumsy. Zach's strengths were that he paid great attention to detail; he became very verbal, and could talk at length and in great detail on different topics; and he had above average intelligence.

Zachary received Early Intervention services from twenty-three to thirty-six months of age. In addition to his Early Intervention services we placed him in a typical pre-school two mornings a week, which he attended with one of his therapists. Four months before he turned three, we began the eligibility process for a special education pre-school placement.

The IEP Process - A Mother Reflects

Although Zachary had made considerable progress since his diagnosis, he still qualified for special education services. I met with the child study team twice after Zach was evaluated, once to go over his test results, and a second time to discuss placement. It was determined that the best placement for him would be a self-contained classroom with up to twelve classified children, with a teacher and two aides. Even though Zachary had been in a nursery school environment already he was initially quite nervous about switching schools. Zach loved reading and fortunately was able to communicate a lot of his anxiety verbally, so I decided to make a social story for him about his new school.

We had a private tour of the facility prior to his entering where I took pictures, and then constructed the story of his upcoming school experience from there. The teachers used visual schedules so that Zach always knew what was happening next, and using that tool seemed to alleviate a great deal of his anxiety. It was evident from testing that Zachary did not have an intellectual disability. His challenges were more in the arenas of social reciprocity and controlling his impulsivity. To that end I worked closely with his teacher to craft specific behavior plans both at home and at school to help him curb his impulses and focus. I had also given considerable input into the creation of his IEP, or Individualized Education Plan. I made certain the goals were specific and quantifiable, and that they covered a variety of areas, such as play skills, socialization skills, academics, hygiene, and focusing skills. Prior to his placement I discussed the make-up of the class he would be attending, ascertaining that there would be both intellectual peers and behavioral role models for him within the classroom. We hashed out which therapies he would receive, and how many times per week he would receive them. Finally, I brought my mother, who is a retired assistant superintendent of schools who handled the special education side, to the meetings with me to help facilitate. Having an advocate at an IEP or related meeting is sometimes necessary to ensure your child does receive what he or she is entitled to- a free and appropriate education.

School and Overall Strategies

Prior to having children, I worked as a regular education teacher for a dozen years in both the Washington D.C., and Fairfax County VA school systems, and as such had a number of students with Asperger's spend part or all of their day in my classroom. There were strategies I employed during my tenure as teacher that became applicable to Zachary's education and have been very helpful to him, such as using a visual schedule to help orient him and prepare him for what comes next. I worked hard to keep to a classroom routine and keep sudden changes to a minimum, and Zach's teachers did the same for him. If there were to be a change in plans I would try to prepare my student with Asperger's in advance. Some of my students benefitted from moving around the room during tests, and sometimes I would permit them to recount information to me orally rather than relying on the written word. I would also allow extra time for tests or projects, and help my students plan projects by using a calendar and breaking down the steps into quantifiable chunks. As much as possible I would keep my directions simple, and be as literal as possible when teaching a new concept to the class. I tried to keep the temperature in the room moderate, and made sure our lighting was constant. I also provided a "safe space" for my students to go when they were feeling overwhelmed. Most importantly, I would remember to encourage my students and reward them whenever their actions merited it. Many of these strategies have also been employed in Zachary's classrooms and have helped him to be successful and productive in school.

Addressing Sensory Issues

I often found with my students with Asperger's that if sensory issues were reduced, they were far more able to learn and contribute to the classroom. To that end, I would try to reduce smells and loud noises as all of these stimuli could be distracting. I never demanded eye contact prior to a conversation, and if possible would allow wait time until I felt I had the student's attention. I tried to reduce clutter in my classroom, and attempted to keep the space in an orderly fashion. If a student was having an issue or meltdown I would employ calming techniques such as counting to ten, squeezing a swoosh ball, or allowing the student to walk around the room or spend a few minutes in the hallway. These strategies have also been particularly successful with my son both at home and at school.

If a big project was coming up, I would work with parents prior to the due date to break the project down into smaller parts with multiple deadlines, then communicate frequently with parents regarding said deadlines. I had a few students who didn't like to write their responses, so I would sometimes permit them to record them orally, act out their answers, or use an art form as an alternative to writing.

Time Management/Organization

Many of the strategies I used in the classroom have also worked with Zachary both at home and academically. Giving my son and my students a frequent heads-up as to how much time is left to accomplish an assignment or task makes them feel more in control, and better able to plan the use of their time. Once again, breaking down tasks into manageable parts has been crucial to the completion of large projects.

Recently, it took me and my son almost a month to complete a science fair project, but we did it in small steps, and managed to avoid being frustrated by the task at hand and with each other. With both my son and my students I have found it imperative to give copious amounts of time for classwork, homework and long-term projects.

When I was a classroom teacher, I insisted my students clean their desks frequently, and with a great deal of cajoling, I insist my son keeps his work area organized as well. I kept labeled bins around the room where children knew to turn in their work, and had many of my students with Asperger's and my neurotypical students color code their folders and binders so they could keep their work for each subject separate and organized.

I encouraged the use of a variety of schedules so my students always knew what was coming next, and kept in frequent contact with parents about upcoming projects and deadlines. One of the most important tools I've used with my son and my students is frequent praise, particularly in situations where they've had to be flexible. Frequent rewards are key.

The Art of Teaching Social Skills

One of the best ways to help a student with Asperger's acclimate to school is to make sure the classroom environment is welcoming, and that differences among students are not only accepted, but celebrated. At home Zach's father and I frequently discuss the many talented individuals in the world who have high-functioning autism, a fact which has made our son proud of who he is and also given him a group with whom to identify.

When helping children with Asperger's grow socially it is imperative to model appropriate social behaviors with other students and with peers.

Pairing students with those who have like interests can facilitate appropriate interaction, but it is important that these children branch out from their preferred topics of interest at times, and they should be rewarded when they do so. For classroom projects I would often form groups that included a child with Asperger's as well as a very socially outgoing peer, which often facilitated friendships between the child with Asperger's and others in the group.

Sometimes, if I felt a child was struggling socially I would invite him or her to lunch in the classroom with me, and we would run through a particular scenario moment by moment. This strategy has worked particularly well with Zach in instances where he had difficulty maintaining a friendship due to his insistence that the conversations go his way. Through modeling he's truly begun to overcome his preference for only talking about topics that interest him.

Students with Asperger's are at considerable risk for bullying, and it's imperative that both teachers and parents keep on the lookout for such behavior. Often the bullying transpires where adult supervision is weakest- hallways, recess, or transportation. It's important that your child or student with Asperger's knows bullying is not acceptable, and that telling an adult is imperative. If the parent or teacher has fostered an atmosphere of acceptance in the home and the classroom, and has celebrated differences, the child will be more likely to seek help.

Finally, most kids enjoy being praised for what they do well. Singling out a child for what they're good at can make other students see him or her in a different way, and perhaps even encourage them to seek the child out. At home we often praise Zach for what we call his "unique world view," which has helped give him the confidence to make new friends as he feels he has something to offer.

The Art and Science of Managing Challenging Behaviors

When it comes to either parenting or teaching a child with or without high-functioning autism, it is important to remember that all behavior is communication, especially tantrums. To effectively parent or teach it is imperative to provide children with the tools to communicate their needs and wants in a positive manner.

In order to be proactive with my son, I have employed behavioral plans for him both at home and in school, and have consulted with him in creating both. Including Zach in the process made him feel like he had ownership of the outcome, and made him more amenable to following the conditions of his "contract." When working with my students I always included them and often their parents in the process, as there often weren't enough rewards at school to keep them motivated. Usually they would comply with the plan because they felt invested in its construction. Behavioral plans are often key in shaping desirable behaviors.

One of the most important components in parenting or teaching a child on the spectrum is teaching children how to self-advocate. In my classroom I used a variety of strategies, such as teaching the child with high-functioning autism to let me know he or she had to spend a few minutes in their "safe place," or gently letting me know they were having anxiety issues prior to a meltdown occurring so I could address the problem. Whenever one of my students was proactive this way I would immediately reward him or her, making certain to give the child lots of praise for making the right choice.

I've taught my son to use deep-breathing techniques to calm himself down before a tantrum, and to come to me if he's feeling overwhelmed. I always make certain to compliment him if he self-advocates for what he needs and avoids a tantrum.

Children with high-functioning autism often need a great deal of downtime, and I made certain to build that time into my lessons with my students as well as provide enough leisure time for my son as well. Being consistent with rules is imperative to promoting good behavior, as is preparing students for their next event. Giving them time to accept a change in schedule can sometimes be the key to avoiding a stressful situation.

Even though many students with Asperger Syndrome or high-functioning autism are usually academically on grade level, some may still require academic adaptations, accommodations, and modifications to be successful in school.

My son is allowed to have extra time on tests, which helps to relieve his anxiety and perform better on exams. Making the appropriate modifications to classwork and schoolwork helped my students maintain a positive attitude toward their academics, and helped them avoid frustration. Sometimes it may be necessary to consult a special education teacher or a BCBA (Board Certified Behavior Analyst) to create the appropriate adaptations.

Finally, whenever possible I've attempted to ignore tantrums (attention-seeking behavior) both from my students and from my child. Acknowledging these behaviors just reinforces that the child must act out to get what he or she wants, and is counter-productive. Teaching self-advocating strategies that he or she can use before losing control promotes positive behavior, and said advocating should always be richly rewarded.

Praising the child with Asperger's for what they are doing right is key to lessening unwanted behaviors and encouraging positive ones (Autism Speaks, 2012).

Transition Plan/Postsecondary Opportunities

While advances have been made to support students with high-functioning autism in the postsecondary arena, unfortunately the vast majority are still underserved. According to the journal of Pediatrics, for youth with an ASD only 34.7% had attended college. More than 50% of youth who had left high school in the past two years had no participation in employment or education, and youth with an ASD had the lowest rates of participation compared with other youth with disability in other categories (Shattuck et al., 2012).

Higher income and higher functional ability were associated with higher adjusted odds of participation in postsecondary employment and education (Shattuck et al., 2012).

Fortunately however there are now more options available for students with high-functioning autism spectrum disorder to pursue a postsecondary education. Securing a good placement for a young adult with autism begins with a sound transition plan.

IDEA and the IEP

Legally the Individuals with Disabilities Education Act (IDEA) entitles all eligible children ages three through twenty-one to a public education, making the states themselves responsible for providing the services to make this happen.

One of the most important goals of the IDEA is to prepare students to live as independently as possible and have gainful employment. The Individualized Education Plan (IEP) is the vehicle through which these goals come to fruition. The IEP includes transition planning and should begin at age fourteen. Services end once the child has left high school.

Creating a Transition Plan: The Challenges

It is important to try and include the child with high-functioning autism in the transition process as much as possible. Soliciting their input as to what they want to do after high school and how they want to be involved in the community will help direct the plan, and the child will be far more invested in accomplishing it than if it were solely constructed by the parents and child study team.

Involvement of a child with high-functioning autism in the IEP process can include "the student writing sections of the IEP for modification and approval at the IEP meeting; co-presenting as an equal member of the IEP team; and/or leading the IEP meeting with support from his or her primary teacher" (Shore, 2004).

Talking about their likes and dislikes, the different ways they learn, and things they're good at as well as things that challenge them is key.

Make certain these discussions occur when your child is ready. Change is often difficult for the child with high-functioning autism, and talking about the future can cause anxiety. If they are ready and willing to discuss plans for the future you will end up with an IEP filled with far more attainable goals.

Meeting with the child study team may seem like the perfect time to highlight your child's accomplishments and downplay their weaknesses, but it is important to remember two things. First, a goal is only accomplished if the child can finish it completely independently- requiring partial prompts to complete a task does not count. Second, the IEP/transition plan is designed to facilitate the development of independent skills- the IEP/transition plan should include as many of these goals as possible, including those that are partially mastered so that they can learn to complete them.

When creating the transition plan the team should keep the following things in mind- "People learn best from other people, like learning how to work in places where other people work; people learn best when the things that they learn are useful- like using the telephone or taking the bus or writing a check; (and) it is important to think about things to learn that will help you become more independent where you live and work right now and where you will live and work in the future" (Allen, 2002).

Ideally, the plan should include goals for some type of employment, and participation in the community at large. It should incorporate goals for a post-secondary education, as well as access to adult services. It should also include both a timeline as to when these goals should be met, and the persons responsible for bringing them to fruition.

Preparing for College

Before an individual with high-functioning autism applies for a post-secondary opportunity it is important to know that IEP diplomas are not recognized by colleges.

The student must have a GED or High School diploma in order to enroll. Many colleges require the ACT or SAT be taken for admission. Sometimes accommodations can be made for taking these exams. If that is possible the paperwork would have to be filed with the school many months prior to the date of the exam. It is imperative not to leave this until the last minute. Last, in order to ease the courseload of the first semester at college sometimes prerequisites can be taken at a local community college and transferred to the accepting college (Autism Speaks, 2013b).

Laws Regarding Post-Secondary Training

It is important to know your rights. According to Section 504 of the Rehabilitation Act, post-secondary programs cannot reject individuals simply because they have a disability. In essence, if you have a disability but you have accomplished what you need to accomplish to get into that program, it is incumbent on the program to give you the supports you need to participate fully in that program.

Selecting a College/Supports

Prior to the process of selecting a school it is important for the student and his or her family to educate themselves about the different types of college programs for students with disabilities. These include but are not limited to:

- Two and four year college or university programs where no specialized courses for students with disabilities are provided, but accommodations are made for disabled students (The Institute for Community Inclusion, 2012).
- Two and four year college or university programs created specifically for students with disabilities only (The Institute for Community Inclusion, 2012).
- Two and four year college or university programs which are separate from the other programs running at these institutions (The Institute for Community Inclusion, 2012).
- Vocational schools (Roberson, Blumberg, and Baker, 2005).

There are a variety of individuals who could be helpful in having a student select a program. Talking to the student's guidance counselor, current or past teachers, and soliciting various autism organizations could help generate a list of colleges and universities which might be appropriate (Autism Speaks, 2013b).

Parents should consider location, cost, admission requirements, campus life and what disability-related supports are available when making your decision (Roberson et al., 2005).

Make certain when visiting the chosen universities or colleges that inquiries are made about kinds of specific school supports for high-functioning autistic students. These supports can include but are not limited to:

- Auditing a course (student may later take the course for credit) (The Institute for Community Inclusion, 2012).
- Making sure a course has no pre-requisites (The Institute for Community Inclusion, 2012).
- More time on tests (Roberson et al., 2005).
- Note-takers (Roberson et al., 2005).
- Assistive Technology (Roberson et al., 2005).
- Preferential seating (Autism Speaks, 2013b).
- Textbook on tape (Autism Speaks, 2013b).
- Tutor who helps student self-advocate and plan for long-term assignments (Roberson et al., 2005).

Pre-Requisite Living Skills/Campus Living

For the high-functioning autistic individual much preparation for a successful experience in a post-secondary placement can be conducted at home. Making sure the student knows how to organize assignments and break them down into chunks over periods of time is crucial (tutors can be hired to facilitate this skill). Personal hygiene skills such as teeth brushing, bathing, shaving, etc. should be mastered, as well as home skills such as how to do laundry. Being confident in money management and using a credit card responsibly is a must as well (Autism Speaks, 2013b).

Creating plans for what to do in an emergency, such as who to contact if the student is locked out of their dorm is important for alleviating anxiety. Making certain the student is comfortable finding his or her way around campus and navigating his or her way home is key as well. Finally, and most importantly, the student should have excellent self-advocating skills so that they can problem-solve. Having a tutor on campus to facilitate those skills can be extremely helpful (Autism Speaks, 2013b).

Prior to attending the college or university the student should know where the Office of Student Services is located on campus. It would also be helpful to know if there are any autism support groups either on campus or nearby as they can provide support. There are groups of high-functioning autistic adults who meet on a regular basis who could be very helpful to a college or university student (Roberson et al., 2005).

Employment Opportunities

As mentioned before, while advances in the postsecondary and employment arenas for students with high-functioning autism have been made, more progress need to occur. According to a survey conducted in the journal Pediatrics published in 2012 "only 55.1% of high-functioning autistic individuals held paid employment during the first 6 years after high school" (Shattuck et al., 2012). A similar study conducted by Taylor and Seltzer suggests a similar low rate of employment (56% in sheltered workshops or day workshops). However they did find that young adults with high-functioning ASD were three times as likely to have daytime activities than those with intellectual disability (Taylor and Seltzer, 2011).

There are in fact however a growing number of companies looking to hire high-functioning autistic individuals for their workforce.

According to the Wall Street Journal, SAP, a Germany-based software company, feels that autistic individuals may outperform neurotypical individuals in some job arenas (Wang, 2014). Aspiritech, a not-for-profit located near Chicago, Illinois, provides training and employment for high-functioning autistic adults. Its program provides training on the technical skills of testing software, as well as basic or “soft” skills necessary to be successfully employed (Autism Speaks, 2013a).

Success in the workplace seems to be determined by having particular skills and accommodations in the work environment.

According to the Autism Society of Minnesota, “since people with ASD have difficulties with social cognition and sensory processing, they initially need a more formalized network of support, structured teaching of tasks, ample time to learn the job, and accommodations for sensory differences ... may be the key(s) to successful employment outcomes.”

Some of the accommodations they suggest include clear job expectations, direct communication, using visuals as an organization tool, assigning a job mentor or coach, and establishing job routines (Autism Society of Minnesota).

Self-Advocacy Skills

As with post-secondary opportunities, it is imperative that individuals with high-functioning autism learn how to self-advocate. Knowing your rights and responsibilities, learning to negotiate with others, and speaking up for yourself are key tools to success in employment. Learning to ask for help to conquer an obstacle is important as well. Often a job coach or mentor can help facilitate in these areas (Autism Speaks, 2013a).

Employment Rights

There are several federal laws that protect disabled individuals from employment discrimination in the workplace. They are the Americans with Disabilities Act of 1990 and the Rehabilitation Act of 1973 (PL93-112).

The Americans with Disabilities Act (ADA) prohibits discrimination based on disability. The ADA requires that a workplace with more than 15 employees must provide a reasonable accommodation for the individual with the disability.

A reasonable accommodation is defined as “any change or adjustment to a job or work environment that permits a qualified applicant or employee with a disability to participate in the job application process, to perform the essential functions of a job, or to enjoy benefits and privileges of employment equal to those enjoyed by employees without disabilities” (Americans with Disabilities Act, 1990).

The Rehabilitation Act was signed into law by President Richard M. Nixon on September 26, 1973. It “prohibits discrimination on the basis of disability in programs conducted by federal agencies, in programs receiving federal financial assistance, in federal employment, and in the employment practices of federal contractors” (Autism Speaks, 2013a). This act afforded many people with disabilities the chance to have an education or be employed.

Finding the Right Type of Job

According to the Autism Speaks, *Employment Tool Kit* (2013a), there are several different types of workplace opportunities available to individuals with high-functioning autism. These include: competitive employment, supported employment, customized employment, and self-employment.

- Customized employment: Either part-time or full-time employment at minimum wage or above. No accommodations or supports are offered.
- Supported employment: A service that helps you find competitive employment in a typical workplace, then provides supports in that workplace.
- Customized employment: This involves talking to the employer about tailoring a job to your skills and needs. It can involve job sharing, where two or more people share tasks around a common goal.
- Self-employment: Creating and running a business.

Preparing for the Job Search

There are a variety of things individuals with high-functioning autism can do to facilitate securing a job. These include but are not limited to a cover letter, resume and preparing for an interview. Some tips from Autism Speaks (2013a) for conducting a job search include:

- Make a list of your strengths and weaknesses. Consider which types of employment best match your strongest skills.
- Talk to a Vocational Rehabilitation counselor about different supports you may be able to get, including help with creating a cover letter, resume, and preparing for an interview. Each state has a Vocational Rehabilitation (VR) agency which provides employment supports to people with disabilities.
- Network with personal contacts as well as using social media.
- Write an excellent cover letter and a comprehensive resume. Be sure to include all necessary contact information in both documents. Make certain to list all internships or prior work experiences in the resume.
- Fill out multiple applications. These may be completed either in person on paper, or online.
- Prepare beforehand for an interview. Dress appropriately, show up early, and make certain to emphasize your strengths not your weaknesses.

Social Skills for the Workplace

Social skills (sometimes referred to as "soft skills") in the workplace are just as important as finding the right job placement. Securing a workplace mentor can be a tremendous asset in both acquiring and practicing this particular skillset. A good mentor can help instruct in ways to ask an employer or co-worker for help, or aid an employee in handling constructive criticism. A high-functioning employee with autism can turn to his or her mentor for tips such as what are appropriate and inappropriate workplace discussions topics, and how to communicate with a team. Good mentors will remind the employee to be punctual at work, and to act professionally at all times (Autism Speaks, 2013a).

Conclusion

Even in the right circumstances, high-functioning autism can present many difficulties to both the individual with the disorder and to their families. However, with patience and the right interventions many of these challenges can be successfully overcome. Whether it is incorporating the correct school supports into the child's IEP, or preparing meticulously to seek postsecondary options or employment, a child or adult with Asperger's can reach his or her goals with some guidance and careful planning. Many people, organizations, and companies have come to see high-functioning autism as a gift. Hopefully the world at large will come to see this unique world view as a gift as well.

References

Allen, W. T. (2002). *It's my choice (2014 reprint)*. Saint Paul, Minnesota: Minnesota Governor's Council on Developmental Disabilities.

Americans with Disabilities Act of 1990, Pub. L. No. 101-336, 104 Stat. 328 (1990).

Autism Society of Minnesota. *Meet the future face of employment: Individuals with autism spectrum disorder in technology fields*. Retrieved from http://mn.gov/mnddc/asd-employment/5a-employment-autism.html.

Autism Speaks (2013a). *Employment tool kit*. Retrieved from http://www.autismspeaks.org/sites/default/files/docs/employment_tool_kit.pdf.

Autism Speaks (2013b). *Postsecondary educational opportunities guide*. Retrieved from http://www.autismspeaks.org/family-services/tool-kits/postsecondary.

Autism Speaks (2012). *Supporting learning in the student with autism*. Retrieved from http://www.autismspeaks.org/sites/default/files/sctk_supporting_learning.pdf.

Roberson, K., Blumberg, R. and Baker, D. (2005). *Keeping it real: How to get the support you need for the life you want* (Chapter 6). Retrieved from http://rwjms.rutgers.edu/boggscenter/projects/keep_real_more.html.

Section 504 of the Rehabilitation Act of 1973, Pub. L. No. 93-112, 34 C.F.R. Part 104 (1973).

Shattuck, P. T., Narendorf, S. C., Cooper, B., Sterzing, P. R., Wagner, M., Taylor, J. L. (2012). Postsecondary education and employment among youth with an autism spectrum diagnosis. *Pediatrics*, 129(6), 1042-1049. http://dx.doi.org/10.1542/peds.2011-2864.

Shore, S. M. (2004). Using the IEP to build skills in self-advocacy and disclosure. In: S. M. Shore (Ed.), *Ask and Tell: Self-Advocacy and Disclosure of People on the Autism Spectrum* (pp. 65-106). Shawnee Mission, KS: Autism Asperger Publishing Company.

Taylor, J. L. and Seltzer, M. M. (May 2011). Employment and Post-Secondary Educational Activities for Young Adults with Autism Spectrum Disorders During the Transition to

Adulthood. *Journal of Autism and Developmental Disorders*, 41(5), 566-574. Abstract retrieved from http://link.springer.com/article/10.1007/s10803-010-1070-3#page-1.

The Greenspan Floortime Approach (2014). *What is floortime?* Retrieved from https://www.stanleygreenspan.com/what-is-floortime/

The Institute for Community Inclusion at University of Massachusetts Boston (2012, October 8). *Postsecondary options for students with disabilities.* Retrieved from http://autismnow.org/in-the-classroom/post-secondary-education/postsecondary-education-options-for-students-with-disabilities/

Wang, S. S. (2014, March 27). How Autism Can Help You Land a Job. *The Wall Street Journal.* Retrieved from http://online.wsj.com/news/articles/SB10001424052702304418404579465561364868556.

Index

A

B

C

D

E

F

G

L

M

N

O

P

Q

R

S